Spirituality

Reiki Guide For aura cleansing and reiki self-healing

(Discovering The Secrets of Aura Cleansing & Self-healing and understanding levels and Acquiring Tips for Meditation)

Karen Penczak

Published by Rob Miles

Karen Penczak

All Rights Reserved

Spirituality: Reiki Guide For aura cleansing and reiki self-healing (Discovering The Secrets of Aura Cleansing & Self-healing and understanding levels and Acquiring Tips for Meditation)

ISBN 978-1-989990-25-4

All rights reserved. No part of this guide may be reproduced in any form without permission in writing from the publisher except in the case of brief quotations embodied in critical articles or reviews.

Legal & Disclaimer

The information contained in this book is not designed to replace or take the place of any form of medicine or professional medical advice. The information in this book has been provided for educational and entertainment purposes only.

The information contained in this book has been compiled from sources deemed reliable, and it is accurate to the best of the Author's knowledge; however, the Author cannot guarantee its accuracy and validity and cannot be held liable for any errors or omissions. Changes are periodically made to this book. You must consult your doctor or get professional medical advice before using any of the suggested remedies, techniques, or information in this book.

Upon using the information contained in this book, you agree to hold harmless the Author from and against any damages, costs, and expenses, including any legal fees potentially resulting from the application of any of the information provided by this guide. This disclaimer applies to any damages or injury caused by the use and application, whether directly or indirectly, of any advice or information presented, whether for breach of contract, tort, negligence, personal injury, criminal intent, or under any other cause of action.

You agree to accept all risks of using the information presented inside this book. You need to consult a professional medical practitioner in order to ensure you are both able and healthy enough to participate in this program.

Table of Contents

INTRODUCTION 1

CHAPTER 1: A LITTLE PAST HISTORY 3

CHAPTER 2: HOW DOES REIKI WORK? 7

CHAPTER 3: HOW CAN I GET A QUALIFIED REIKI PRACTITIONER? 12

CHAPTER 4: HOW TO PRACTICE HEALING OTHERS 30

CHAPTER 5: EXPLORE THE DIFFERENT TYPES OF REIKI 46

CHAPTER 6: LEARNING REIKI 50

CHAPTER 7: REIKI TREATMENTS. 55

CHAPTER 8: REIKI SESSIONS: WHAT TO EXPECT 64

CHAPTER 9: BASIC ENERGY ANATOMY 71

CHAPTER 10: HOW TO PRACTICE REIKI ON YOURSELF 83

CHAPTER 11: BENEFITS OF CRYSTAL FOR REIKI 97

CHAPTER 12: SUN ANCON CHI MACHINE....................... 116

CHAPTER 13: HEALTH IMPROVEMENT............................ 134

CHAPTER 14: LEVELS OF REIKI.. 151

CHAPTER 15: REIKI STONES 158

CHAPTER 16: REIKI MASSAGE FOR STRESS REDUCTION . 166

CHAPTER 17: THREE PILLARS OF MODERN REIKI............ 173

CONCLUSION.. 191

Introduction

The universe, most especially planet earth is blessed with various gift from God which are most of the time left untapped by human being. We know of Electrical Electronics Energy

being used to power electronics, Energy of gravity pulling downward and keeping object stationed to the earth, that of magnetism which is of attraction between two or more objects and radiation which is the transmission and emission of energy in the form of particles or waves through an atmosphere or through any material. From western knowledge, our body house most of these energies which are significant basis of human physical existence.

Generally, people are looking for ways to get eased-off of stress developed in our body through daily activities. But finding the right medicine to help achieve this has been a tiring task since a very long time. With this book you will be able to help yourself and others who might be in need of stress relieve.

Reiki is being defined and re-explained in most chapters of this book, which will allow you have a better grasp of the meaning of Reiki.

I'm positive you will be left astonished learning or using this healing techniques.

Chapter 1: A Little Past History

One more fascinating beginning makes use of the identified Mikao Usui that was in enhancement to being a Buddhist Clergyman that was interested in the trainings of Jesus. Usui transformed to Buddhism to locate responses. Due to the fact that of his globe takes a trip looking for solutions of the recovery course Usui is the one that brought Reiki to the Western Globe Center.

Reiki is thought about a spiritual technique that was created by Mikao Usui. On Usui's remembrance rock there is an engraving explaining that he showed Reiki to over 2000 individuals in his life time. Usui established the Reiki Ryoho Gakkai which equates as the Usui's Spiritual Power Treatment Culture; a Japanese culture of Japanese Reiki masters. We could claim that Usui rediscoverd and also created the old techniques of Reiki for the globe to make use of.

Usui researched at holy place college and also proceeded his Buddhist education and learning till he ended up being a zaike or lay Tendai clergyman. He proceeded to examine his entire life as well as his various other researches consisted of; record, medication, Buddhism, Christianity, Taoism as well as psychology. Considering that of his origins Usui was likewise increased samurai especially aiki jutsu.

In enhancement to being a Tendai Buddhist, it was stated that Usui likewise exercised Shugenja likewise recognized as Shugendo. Shugenja or Shugendo is referred to as a Japanese spartan shamanistic method including aspects of both Shintoism and also Buddhisim.

Usui started the Reiki Ryoho Gakkai which equates as the Usui's Spiritual Power Treatment Culture; a Japanese culture of Japanese Reiki masters. It was Usui in the

Zen abbeys in Japan after examining the Sanskrit works that he felt he discovered the solution of recovery. We could claim that Usui rediscoverd and also created the old methods of Reiki for the globe to utilize.

Since of his globe takes a trip looking for responses of the recovery course Usui is the one that brought Reiki to the Western Globe Leading edge.

Reiki is thought about a spiritual method that was created by Mikao Usui. Mikao Usui was birthed in was birthed in 1865. On Usui's remembrance rock there is an engraving explaining that he instructed Reiki to over 2000 individuals in his life time.

Shintoism affected Usui, which is a typical Japanese belief that was affected by the Chinese previous to its creation in Japan. Usui himself utilized "jamon" which are spells as well as necromancies in his trainings that obtained from both Shintoism as well as Taoism.

The Japanese word Reiki in Shinjitai Japanese or Katana indicates strange atmosphere/spiritual power which is acquired from the Chinese word lingqi significance spiritual impact (of points such as hills). No matter of the words connected with the word Reiki it steams down to life pressure as well as global power, which is spiritual in nature.

Chapter 2: How Does Reiki Work?

Now that you know what Reiki is, the next step is to find out just how it works. Essentially, Reiki involves manipulation of your life force energy but isn't the actual life force energy. Confused yet? That's perfectly fine. Let's look at it in a different way and see if I can't clear up your confusion.

Your heart works through the contraction and relaxation of muscles stimulated by an electrical charge that keeps your heartbeat smooth and regular. If something is out of kilter in your heart and the electrical charges don't work right, a doctor may prescribe medications or surgically install tiny machines that assist in keeping those synapses between the muscles of your heart firing properly. Those are the pacemakers or defibrillators you hear about people having implanted. But if your heart stops, a 'crash cart' or defibrillator paddles are used to start it again by sending a jolt of electricity from an outside source through it.

The Energy Meridians

Your body at the core has energy meridians that flow through it. The following image is a diagram of how energies run through your body and the directions these energy currents run. The different meridian channels affect different portions of your body. The meridian line that runs from the crown of your head touches all of the other channels producing a conjunction where two lines intersect. Which is why simply following the main line from crown to core (the base of your spine) will allow you to smooth out those auxiliary lines at the same time.

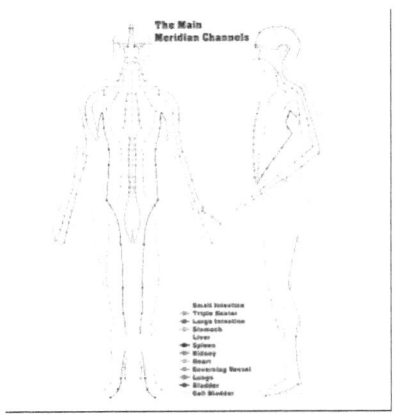

Reiki works on that same principle since it is usually performed by a practitioner on a patient. The role of patient is pretty self-explanatory, while the practitioner is the outside source that is smoothing out those rapids in your life force energy we talked about earlier. Those ripples, knots, and blocks in the energy flow is what's causing you to feel unwell.

Life Force sustains you

Therapists who practice Reiki say that you are alive because of the life force flowing through you. This life force moves along paths or channels in your body that are commonly called chakras, meridians, or nadis. This life force runs through all the organs and cells of your body providing nourishment and support for all the functions carried out within each system.

The life force in your body can affect your health in both positive and negative ways through the thoughts and feelings you have about yourself. More specifically, the feelings about yourself in your subconscious mind that you may not be aware of having. The negative thoughts or feelings you have about yourself will cause ripples, eddies and knots in the flow of that energy causing you to feel physically unwell.

What a Reiki practitioner does is to introduce *positive* energy into those disturbed areas to 'charge' them to a point where the negative energies break up and just fall away. The slow, harmful vibrations become faster, healthier vibrations that help you feel better. When that happens, the positive energies used by the therapist smooth out your natural energies and whatever problem you were having will ease and finally disappear.

Reiki practitioners believe and will tell you that *they* are not guiding the healing but that the energy within you is doing what it already knows you need. The practitioner is just the conduit the energy is using to get past the blockages, or rapids, to get to where it needs to go. Therefore, even if Reiki doesn't work as well as you think it should for whatever problem you were, or are, having – it's not going to make the problem worse! That's reassuring, isn't it?

Come on! Let's see how Reiki can help you to relax.

Chapter 3: How Can I Get A Qualified Reiki Practitioner?

Ask a friend who's doing Reiki.

Although today people are used to receiving healthcare from professionals, Reiki does not need this. To receive Reiki training no special experience or qualifications are needed. Reiki was created as a folk healing practice, and you might want to receive Reiki from your friend if you have a friend who is trained, and who regularly practices with himself. If you are happy with this experience, you can go on with your friend or contact the Reiki master of your friend.

Find a medical practitioner who does Reiki.

You can consider a Reiki practitioner in private or a healthcare facility if you do not have a friend who does Reiki. Reiki practitioners have become more and more skilled in private practice and provide Reiki in health-care settings in recent years. However, more medical institutes use Reiki in their treatment model. More than 800 U.S. states, according to the American Hospital Association. In 2007, Reiki was provided by hospitals as part of their hospital services. The Reiki Research Center website lists 71 hospitals, medical clinics and hospice programmes, in which Reiki is a standard medical care facility. As part of their patient care, many health care professionals and nurses offer Reiki either through integrating Reiki contact into routine care or through long Reiki sessions. A hospital stay may provide the first chance to have a Reiki session.

Word of the mouth is a good strategy to locate a doctor. Complementary therapy practitioners locally (for example, acupuncture, shiatsu, reflexology, massage, herbalism, homeopathy, etc.) usually know each other by their reputation and sometimes share offices or cross-references.

Look in your community.

You could try looking at group newsletters in Yoga Studios and health food stores as with seeking a Reiki practitioner. Moreover, your local hospital can have an integrative or complementary medicine service. Because Reiki is used by many to cope with chronic illness, a community resource list or even the sponsor of a reiki clinic may include any local organization providing services to individuals with diseases, such as cancer, HIV, fibromyalgia and diabetes.

How do I assess their skills and qualifications?

How can you measure qualifications once you find a Reiki practitioner? What are you supposed to look for? As the Reiki profession has originated not from formal healthcare programs but from a grassroots movement, many different views and methods of practice have been established without guidance and no pattern of training or treatment is universal in all practice types.

Although Reiki masters often give certificates to their students, they do not support education standards agreed throughout the Reiki community. Therefore, the possession of a credential does not guarantee thorough training for the practitioner. To assess training and experience, you need to ask some specific questions.

What are some questions I ought to ask?

When you decide to seek Reiki from a practitioner, search for someone who has been educated and who has extensive experience in providing Reiki to others. The most important thing is that the practitioner performs Reiki every day since this is how he establishes a relationship with Reiki and deepens his / her understanding.

Professionals usually produce a brochure and/or website that outlines their requirements for training and practice. Look for answers to the questions below and any other questions you might have:

What is the level of training (first or second degree or master's degree Reiki)?

You can get Reiki from someone at any level of Reiki training. You need a second-degree practitioner if you are looking for distant healing. You need a Reiki master, if you want to learn how to practice Reiki yourself.

Where have you been trained?

It gives you an insight into how long the individual performs, even if it depends on how much she practices. For example, someone who practiced Reiki five years ago but does not use it often would be less attractive than someone who uses it every day.

How long have the lessons been?

Eight to 12 hours for the first degree and another 8 to 12 hours for the second degree course provides time for training as well as practical learning in the classroom. Classes given in a 2-3 day format offer more time for training.

For second graduates or masters in Reiki: Have you been trained at each level in separate lessons and if so, how far are the classes apart?

The second degree training preferably took place a minimum of three to six months after the first degree course. This would give the practitioner ample time before learning the more involved and abstract, distant healing techniques. Some Reiki masters require at least 1 year between Reiki grades 1 and 2.

The minimum required is to practice an extra one to two years before becoming a Reiki master. Traditional Reiki masters often require that students have even more experience.

What is your clinical experience, to whom and for how many years have you been treated?

It is reasonable to expect years of expertise, not only for families and friends, but also for people beyond the social circles of the practitioner who have varying levels of health and wellness. Some Reiki practitioners may have worked as volunteers in the Reiki Hospital before beginning their own practice.

How are you going to describe Reiki?

For a specialist, this should not be a difficult question to answer. You don't want to believe he or she has never before been worried about this. The practitioner should be able to clearly and authoritatively describe the practice.

Be careful about practitioners who claim that they are healing or who disregard traditional healthcare.

The answer to this question is often when the practitioner becomes aware of the person and when you feel comfortable with him or her.

Describe the duration and the fee of your sessions.

You would want someone who explains the system clearly and how it is structured so you have an idea of what to expect. (On your initial appointment an experienced professional confirms this information.) Ask if the practitioner uses techniques other than Reiki in the session and decide whether you want Reiki. (Consider: if you don't have only a Reiki session, how can you know whether it is Reiki that is great for you?)

Do you Practice Reiki on yourself daily?

This is the most important issue. Good for someone who practices Reiki self-care every day, as this is how practitioners continue to develop and deepen their relationship with Reiki.

NOTE: If the information above is not readily available, a prospective practitioner can be interviewed briefly by telephone or via email. This inquiry will be accepted by a reputable practitioner.

What is the cost of Reiki?

Generally, Reiki is only paid if it is included in the treatment as part of routine care during a hospital stay, such as physical therapy, acupuncture and palliative care covered by the insurance, or if it is given by a nursing or a licensed health care professional. If you are visiting a Reiki practitioner, plan to pay out of your pocket.

The cost of a session varies and this is dependent on the provider's experience, whether they are professionals working in the full-time public practice and the local economy, but the cost of a session is generally up to $50-75. Reiki students may offer Reiki for lower costs as they gain clinical experience and Reiki clinics or community groups are available for donations or low fees, where sessions are available.

IN A STANDARD REIKI SESSION, WHAT CAN I EXPECT?

There is, in some respects, no standard Reiki session-no protocol or time-length. Reiki can be run by anyone who is qualified, who can be a specialist, a freind or family member, healthcare provider, or even you yourself if you have been trained in Reiki. In addition, there is no typical setting: a quiet spot is preferable, but Reiki can be done wherever, regardless of what else happens to or around the receiver. A Reiki-trained practitioner's contact moments can provide support in an acute or emergency situation, such as onset of influenza or after an accident or surgery.

This segment discusses what to expect from someone, a practitioner or a friend who took at least first degree practice, in a complete or updated full session.

Who Should I See?

Take time to find and choose a practitioner (professional or friend) with whom you feel comfortable and who meets your standards to ensure you have the best experience possible. (But a friend may not have the same degree of experience as a professional, receiving Reiki from a friend can be a special experience if you're comfortable and open to each other).

You'll want someone who clearly describes the way and how he or she structures the session, so you have an idea what to expect. Your actual therapy experience is very personal, but understanding what the doctor will do next helps you relax.

Reiki Environment

A quiet environment is always desirable where you are not disturbed. Registered Reiki practitioners have a dedicated room or are experienced when making house calls. We sometimes play soft music as a way to mask ambient noise during the session, but let your practitioner know if you want silence.

Those that undergo Reiki in a hospital, hospice, nursing home or in another healthcare facility, but might have a shorter session (15 to 20 minutes). Most of the sessions are between.

Is there any Intake Process?

Many practitioners have intakes, particularly if the practitioner has other healthcare or manual therapy practice, such as massage. Nevertheless, because Reiki has originated rather than a health care technique as a traditional tradition, most Reiki practitioners actively resist the kind of intake typical in health care. You may be requested to sign an authorization form.

The practitioner explains the process and asks whether you have specific needs. Ensure to let the doctor know whether you have a health condition that could affect your lying flat on your back or forehead or if you have touch-sensitive areas. Practitioners can ask for permission to touch in a hospital or other healthcare setting.

What Does Reiki Session Consist of?

A complete Reiki session is given to the fully clothed client who sits comfortably in a chair on a treatment table.

Reiki is generally offered through light, non-invasive hands, which are placed and held in a number of places on the torso head and front and back. The hands should never be inappropriate or intrusive or pressure should be exerted.

Further placing on the limbs can be done if necessary (for example, if there is an injury or surgical scar), and this is routinely done by some practitioners. If necessary, the Reiki practicer can hold her hands off the body (e.g. in front of an open burn or wound), and some practicers always offer Reiki in this way.

What Could I Experience?

"I think I've fallen asleep." "I can't believe how hot you have your hands!" "I feel so relaxed than even after a massage." "My headache is gone." These are some things that some people typically say after a Reiki sitting.

Reiki's experience is personal, shifting, and sometimes very subtle. People often experience heat in the hands of the practitioner, but at times the hands of the practitioner are cool. Some common sensations are slight pulsations, where the hands of the practitioner are positioned and waves of pulsations cascading all over the body.

People often comment on how comfortable Reiki's experience is. An interesting study indicated that recipients frequently think that they are at a threshold state of consciousness, simultaneously aware of their world and deeply drawn into it. Some people fall into a deep, sleepy trance. Reiki's experience is sometimes dramatic, while the first session can be un-accidental for others in particular, although they feel better later on. The most common experience is almost instant a feeling of deep relaxation and stress release.

Reiki is cumulative, and yet people who don't remember much usually have deeper experiences as they start. Besides Reiki's immediate experience, you can see other changes that continue to unfold over the course of the day: perhaps strong digestion, a more centered, more balanced, less reactive feel, and a deeper sleep that night.

During The Session, What Should I Do?

When you have taken the time to select a reputable practitioner with whom you have friendships, what can you do to make your Reiki experience comfortable? Not a lot, but here are some suggestions:

If you have music you really enjoy and relax, take it to your session and ask the practitioner to play it. Whether you choose, you can also ask for silence.

Use the rest room in advance of your session to sit comfortably.

Especially if you're timid about being touched, ask your practitioner before beginning to show you your hands so that your expectations are very clear.

Before you begin, let the practitioner know your needs. For instance, if you have trouble breathing and lie flat, say so. Or if you've recently had surgery, note that you don't want to be treated where the wound is tender (the doctor can float her hand here). It may not be possible to lie on your stomach if you are pregnant or have digestive problems. Inform your doctor.

You would feel more relaxed as the session progresses. If you are uncomfortable, you can always change your spot. Be sure to ask anything, such as additional support under your knees or blankets that will increase your comfort.

This is your particular time and the doctor will support you.

It's a wonderfully passive experience to receive Reiki. Don't try to relax, just relax with Reiki. As the session continues, the condition will change very naturally. In the meantime, feel free to dream, enjoy the music, or just watch your breath or therapy sensations.

What's Happen After the Session?

Don't expect a cure because Reiki doesn't. Many clinicians may make sensible aftercare recommendations such as drinking water and meeting the needs of your body.

While people usually leave a Reiki session feeling refreshed, they often feel tired during the night. This is not seen as an adverse reaction, but rather as a natural healing reaction of the body. People also say that they are calm and mentally aware and that after Reiki they sleep well.

How Many Sessions Should I Get?

The doctor may recommend a number of sessions. Four sessions are a standard guideline and give you time to evaluate the benefits you receive. Speak to your doctor how to arrange the sessions better for your needs and schedule.

Reiki practitioners often recommend four sessions over four days in the presence of the serious health challenge. The same practitioner does not need to give these.

Chapter 4: How To Practice Healing Others

Eventually you will become skilled enough and practiced enough to not only use your reiki techniques on yourself, but also on others. There are a few things to note that are different when it comes to working with others' energy.

Consent

An absolute crucial element of practicing reiki is the intent of the practitioner and that they have only a healing mindset. Of course, without this element one is simply not performing reiki. While I am sure that you reading this book have nothing but positive intentions and expectations in regard to how you will use your newfound skills, it is necessary to reinforce the importance of utter respect, consent, and privacy. The laying on of hands is a powerful force, obviously, which is why you are interested in learning about it. With that great power comes an absolute responsibility to use it wisely, safely, and respectfully.

Because reiki requires the master to either put hands physically on or very near to a person's body, it is important to check in with that person before doing so. Every person is different, and while there are certainly areas of another person's body that may seem like obvious private spaces, each person may have their own areas that are especially sensitive or off limits. You should respect these boundaries at all times, and be communicative about your intentions.

Of course, every part of the body can benefit from the treatment of the laying on of hands, and that includes areas that are sensitive or people are uncomfortable with another person touching. This is not a problem at all. It is most important to be professional and respectful, because there are ways to still treat these areas while following limits of each individual.

A great way to go about ensuring everyone will be comfortable throughout the session is to begin with a conversation.

As is the case with all physical contact, you should ask permission before beginning. Before doing anything else or even touching the person, you should have an explicit, clear, informed, enthusiastic conversation about what you plan on doing and whether or not that is acceptable to them. Explaining what you plan on doing will help them have a better understanding of what they can expect, and therefore will allow them to give more informed consent. This also means that you should explain to them that although they may give you permission now, they are always able to remove their consent at any time and for any reason. It is reassuring to them if you check in frequently throughout the session to continue obtaining consent and validating the interaction. As a practitioner, you should do everything you can to make them feel comfortable in being honest about their boundaries, but you should also emphasize their ability and freedom to say no, and that you will never pressure them into accepting or doing anything they are uncomfortable with. Along that same note, you should be cognizant enough of their body language to be able to tell if they are anxious, uncomfortable, or keeping something inside.

The amazing thing about reiki is its omnipotent knowledge of what needs to be healed, whether the practitioner is aware of it or not. For this reason, it is not even necessary to put your hands on or near any areas they are not comfortable with. Obviously there is the option of simply hovering your hands over the area, but even if that is not something they want, you can place your hands in a different area and focus the energy to travel to any other area. By focusing on where you intend the life force to travel to will be enough to increase flow to those spots. Another option would be to have the person place their own hands on that area, and then you can either place your hands over theirs, hover your hands over theirs, or simply use their own hands to channel the energy to that area, using themselves as a conduit.

Another aspect of them giving consent to you not only has to deal with you touching them, but also simply them agreeing that you can use reiki on them. Because the art of using the universal life force is not actually something you possess and are transferring to another, but simply using your knowledge to invite them to be healed with the energy they already possess and is pulsing in, through, and around them. It is not an art that you can decide to use to heal another. You are not in control of it or the judge of how to use it. It is present with or without you. You are simply attempting to channel it. For that reason, the only way for it to work is for the person receiving it to give permission to do so. Even if you have the best of intentions and all you want to do is help another, it will not work to attempt to control or force something on another person, even if that thing is healing. So when it comes to a session in person with the other, this consent can and should be given explicitly.

However, as you progress into the second degree of training, you will become able to do distance healing. In this instance, the recipient may or may not be aware that you are attempting to perform reiki upon and through them. What does this mean for getting consent? Well, it means that rather than requiring explicit consent before you start, it means that you will ask the universe and their unconscious for consent to work with their energy. Because of reiki's all-knowing presence, it will never encroach upon a person who is not consenting, either consciously or unconsciously. The way this happens is not by you performing reiki on another, but instead by offering what can be accepted. They neither cannot nor will not be able to take more than they need or want, nor will the omnipotent universe energy force it upon a not receiving recipient.

This does not mean you should necessarily ignore or bypass the needs of people for whom you cannot explicitly ask for consent. In fact, by using distance healing you can feel empowered to offer your services to any and all beings in need. The wonderful thing is that it will only penetrate to those who are accepting of it. This receptivity may or may not be conscious or explicit on their part, and for that reason, your efforts may very well reach their intended targets by simply them having an open mind and heart to it. All of this is also applicable to not only other people, but also animals, plants, and other objects. Although not all other beings speak verbally, the same concept will apply to all of them.

Your Ability

Of course you will want to keep the recipient in the forefront of your mind when performing reiki on another person. However, it is important to also keep in mind your ability and comfort level during the session. Depending on how long you plan on spending time with the person, a full hour is a very common amount of time to spend with one person in a single session. That means you need to mentally and physically prepare for spending sixty minutes serving another.

Not only should they be comfortable during the session, but you also need to be comfortable. What does that mean for you? It means that in setting them up for the session, you should consider whether you want to or physically can stand or sit for the duration of it. For some reiki masters, they prefer to have the recipient lying down. In order for the master to best serve them, it is easier if they have a table to lay on much like a massage table. That brings the recipient up to a height so that the master does not have to bend for long periods of time, as well as providing a comfortable surface for the recipient as they lie either face up or face down. With a table, the master can both stand as well as sit at a comfortable level to lay hands. However, you might prefer for them to be seated upright in a chair. That way you can stand without much bending and even sit alongside them.

Expectations

For a person who has never experienced reiki before, or if they are simply new to your practice, you will want to give them some information to prepare themselves for what they are about to experience. Even for someone with whom you have been working for some time, every day and session will be different, so it is also good to set expectations from day-to-day with regular recipients.

As was discussed in the previous chapter, you will want to share with them they ways they will want to prepare beforehand, such as being well rested and hydrated, among other things. You will also want to let them know what type of clothing to wear.

At the beginning of your session, you will also want to go over what you plan on doing and getting consent, as was already discussed. After you have done that, you will want to prepare them for what they might experience during the session. Some of the most common reactions and feelings that occur throughout the body during sessions include: tingling sensations, heat, cold, muscle spasms, relaxation, falling asleep, itching, stomach growling, and others. There can also be some psychological reactions possible, including: seeing or visualizing flashes of color or light, memories rushing in, flashes of a past life, strong emotions coming up, and even feeling the sensation of touching or movement where there is none.

All of that is to say, these are simply a few of the things that they may experience. They may experience many other things not listed. It is also very possible that they do not seem to notice experiencing anything at all! All of these are perfectly fine, and none of them are indicative of the effectiveness of the reiki session. More of a reaction does not necessarily mean more happened, and no reaction does not mean nothing worked.

It is also very common and possible that they will have some of these or other reactions in the hours, days, or even weeks following their session. Because the session is not a one-time occurrence of energy flowing, but it is in fact simply initiating the universe to continue focusing its life force through this specific area of a person, it is expected that changes will occur after the session. Your goal is not to change someone once right then, but instead to begin an ongoing flow. What is also most impressive and interesting to share with your client is that it is actually themselves who are doing the healing. Therefore, it is not delayed responses to your reiki session with them that they will experience, but it is truly their own bodies having learned how to use reiki through themselves and for themselves!

Remove Yourself

As you are performing a service via the art of laying hands, it should be a given that you would not be the focus of such acts of service. However, whenever it comes to reiki especially, you are simply a vessel through which the universe's life force travels through. It is not you that is doing the healing. It is not you that is finding the areas of need. It is not you that is deciding what needs to be done. The utmost energy is already there and able to travel to where it is most needed. You are merely a conduit to encourage the other person to get their own energy flowing freely. You are allowing the life force to flow through to another person, but it exists and can be manipulated with or without your presence.

This is not a cautionary tale in order to denigrate your ability or sense of purpose. Not at all. In fact, it is merely a reminder to humble yourself in front of the all-knowing and all-encompassing life force that is the universe around us. The power is too great to think any mere mortal is control it or be its equal. This should not be a depressing fact, but instead an awe-inspiring; one that reinforces the importance of your work. To assist others in becoming masters of their own energy and becoming one with the universe that lives within and around themselves is a truly magnificent gift and service.

One aspect of removing yourself from the process means that you should not become a channel for their negative energy or blockages. The art of reiki is not a zero-sum game; just because the other person has a restriction they want to be healed does not mean that you need to take it upon yourself in order to free them of it.

In fact, it is not even your energy that you are using to help them heal. You are a channel for their own energy, which is actually that of the Universe. You cannot and will not deplete your own reserves or source. In fact, you should not even have a feeling of being tired or emotionally depleted from performing a session on another. For this reason, it is very unlikely that you will experience this, but under rare circumstances, it has been known to occur.

It is very common and understandable that as a healer, you have a deep vested interest in helping another person. This need to be of service and heal others can often feel like an overwhelming sense of purpose, and to not fulfil those duties can leave you feeling lost and underwhelming, or like you are not living up to your potential. While these are noble and completely understandable desires, this shows a deep attachment to expectations that are not helpful. As part of your reiki training, you should be focusing on turning inward and growing in your own personal development, especially when it comes to deep seated issues. While this particular issue has most likely served you very well in your past or in other areas of your life, it is important to recognize how this can and will negatively impact your life and reiki. What is most likely happening is to do with a level of empath healing that occurs at the same time as a reiki session, and it is being misattributed to the reiki. If this happens, you should seek assistance from another reiki master, and attempt to work through any empath boundary deficiencies you may have.

Another important aspect of removing yourself from the practice has to due to fulfilling others' expectations. Because this art cannot be fully explained scientifically as of yet, that leaves some people skeptical and requiring certain benchmarks be met for them to believe or understand it. These people may tell you explicitly that this is the case, but in a lot of cases, it may simply be a story you are telling yourself about how other people are thinking without saying it. This means you are assuming how the other person is feeling, assuming that it is negative or skeptical about reiki, and therefore you feel the need to somehow prove or perform a certain way in order to justify the art of reiki to a nonbeliever. This is a manifestation of trying to soothe your ego by justifying your practice to another person, and it is neither necessary nor helpful to the art of healing.

Chapter 5: Explore The Different Types Of Reiki

Usui Reiki is the original form of Reiki. But, over the years, there have been several branches that have stemmed from it due to cultural and religious adaptations. There are specific methods of meditation and also special symbols for each form of Reiki that have developed over the years. In this chapter, we will discuss the most common types of Reiki that are practiced in the world today:

Usui Reiki

This is the original and the first form of Reiki that has been practiced all over the world. It was rediscovered and brought back to the modern world in the year 1922 by Mikao Usui. Dr. Chujiro Hayashi studied Usui Reiki extensively and passed it on to several students of his. One of his most noted students, Hawayo Takata took this practice to the West. The changes made by these two influential Reiki practitioners has led to the several systems of Reiki that we know of today.

Karuna Reiki

This form of Reiki finds its origins in Hinduism and Buddhism. In fact, the name comes from the Sanskrit word "Karuna" which is used in both the religions. Karuna means compassion and this form of Reiki is based mostly on the Universal Compassion concept of Buddhism. William Lee Rand developed this system of Reiki. He founded the International Center for Reiki Training. The goal of this form of Reiki is to heal others and alleviate their suffering with Reiki.

Rainbow Reiki

This is one of the most recent practices of Reiki that was developed in the early 90s. Its founder, Walter Lubek based the practice on the teachings of Reiki master Hawayo Takata. It was introduced to the

West in the year 1937. Several techniques like chakra work and cleaning of the karma have been developed in this practice of Reiki. They use the assistance of the Inner Child and the Higher Self within each individual to make this practice of Reiki more powerful. You can use the positive power of these two states of your being to harness the actual power of Reiki.

Kundalini Reiki

This form of Reiki focuses on raising your energy for healing through the root chakra as opposed to other practices that encourage you to release this energy from the crown chakra. This activation of the Kundalini is possible with regular practice of Yoga that helps clear blockages in the chakra. When you are able to raise your Kundalini, you feel at complete ease with yourself. Happiness and strength are derived from this form of Reiki. Ole Gabrielsen first developed this form of Reiki. It gained more and more momentum as the popularity of Yoga increased world over.

You can practice any form of Reiki that suits you the best. Each one has its own philosophy and methods of practice. You may be introduced to one form of Reiki and may even move on to other practices depending upon what makes you feel positive and energized.

Chapter 6: Learning Reiki

Now that you are familiar with the chakras, auras, symbols, and the philosophy behind the Reiki practice, you can get started on how to practically learn it. Your first step in the learning as well as practicing of Reiki is finding a facility where you can derive attunement. This is the process during which the Reiki master transfers energy to their student.

During this process, the heart; the crown; and also the palm chakras; are all opened between the student and the Reiki source. In this process, guides are in attendance as well as spiritual beings who implement the process. There are even some people who have reported some experiences during this process that involve receiving messages of a personal nature; visions; healing; and also life experiences from way back in their past. Sometimes, soon after undergoing the process of receiving a

Reiki attunement, there have been students reporting their psychic sensitivity increasing and they experience psychic abilities after this process.

You should be aware that Reiki attunement is able to start a cleansing process that will affect the physical body as well as the mind and emotion. Toxins stored in the body may be released and thought patterns that are no longer useful may be eradicated. The process of purification is recommended before you take on the process of attunement.

There are several ways that you can prepare for your attunement. The first step recommended is to refrain from eating meat, fowl or fish for three days prior to your ceremony. The three foods mentioned can contain growth hormones and antibiotics that will throw off your balance and make it sluggish. The next step is considering water or juice fast for one or even three days; of course, only if your health allows. Be sure to check with a medical professional if you don't know. Other foods to avoid include sweets and chocolate for three days prior to your attunement.

When it comes to beverages, avoid anything that has caffeine in it as much as possible. They create imbalances in your body; specifically within your endocrine and also nervous system. Ensure you avoid partaking of any caffeine beverage on the day of your attunement. Do not drink any alcoholic beverages for three days before your attunement.

If you take any type of drugs that do not keep you alive, such as smoking, then do not take them the day of your attunement.

In order to balance your spiritual and mental state, meditate for an hour a day for at least a week before the ceremony. Use a style that you already know or spend this time in silence in order to become more in touch with your inner peace as well as innner soul. Bring down your TV watching time; listening to music, and even reading newspapers. You want to be emotionally balanced; and yet all these are undertakings that can put you off balance. In fact, it would be advisable that you go for a quiet walk and spent time with nature to get some exercise rather than watched television or did something sedentary.

To prepare yourself emotionally for this change in your life, you should pay more attention to the subtleness in people and nature around you. Release all fear; jealousy; hatred; anger; worry; and even anxiety, by making a place within you and around you that you are comfortable and at peace in. Remember that you are receiving more than just attunement. You are becoming part of a group of people using Reiki to heal themselves and others, and they're working together to heal the planet.

Whenever you are in doubt, recall that you are receiving help from guides and spiritual beings that work towards attaining your goals. Even while you are not religious, it is helpful to be ready to open yourself to some higher spiritual energy and experience.

Now that you know what to expect when it comes to attunement, let's move forward. After you are through with attunement, it is great to be able to learn from Reiki Master. Practically, though, it is not always possible. Don't fret; there are plenty of guides out there that will teach you the different positions and techniques when you are practicing. I am going to go ahead and explain some of those techniques to you to give you a better understanding of Reiki.

Chapter 7: Reiki Treatments.

PERFORMING THE TREATMENT:

It is important not to absorb any of the cat's physical and emotional distress during the treatment. To protect yourself, clearly set your intent, before beginning the treatment, so that you will not take on any negative energy from the cat. If you do feel that you have taken some negative energy, use your hands to "sweep" down your arms and body to brush it off into the ground for recycling.

It is also very important that you take a "no expectations" approach to the treatment process and to its results. Do not personalize them – even if it is your own cat that you are working on. Stay neutral. Understand that the flow of Reiki energy will have "peaks and valleys" during the treatment. Reiki provides only the amount of energy that the cat is willing to accept.

I like to begin each treatment by softly asking that, "The Reiki energy be used only for (the cat's name) greatest and highest good." If your are a Reiki Level II practitioner or a Reiki Master-Teacher, you can draw in the air or visualize any of the Reiki symbols that you are qualified to use, activating them by saying their names as a mantra three times for each one used. Then simply intend that Reiki begin flowing and it will.

If the Reiki energy seems to be lessening shortly after you begin the treatment, the cat may be evaluating the energy to make sure that it is comfortable with it. Continue the treatment, but be alert for signs of acceptance or rejection from the cat.

HANDS-ON REIKI:

Although most cats prefer to receive Reiki from a distance because of their sensitivity to the energy's intensity, cats that are

familiar with you may be comfortable with the Hands-on approach described here. In such cases, you may even be able to give them Reiki while petting or stroking them.
A receptive cat may be still or may move around some during the treatment, exposing different parts of its body to the energy.

Which body parts of the cat that you can directly place your hands on for treatment will depend on where you can physically reach on the cat's body, where the cat will allow you to touch, and where it is safe to touch (when injury or illness may result in body areas that are too sensitive to touch). Remember, however, that Reiki will flow to wherever it is most needed when you do a Hands-on treatment.

You do not need to follow a specific pattern of hand placements; let the cat's behavior guide you. A good generic placement of hands would be on the cat's shoulders and upper chest or to start with hands on its shoulders and then gradually working down its spine to the base of its tail. Treat the cat's head last as many cats don't like receiving energy there. If the cat becomes deeply relaxed, don't disturb them by changing the position of your hands.

As with any Reiki treatment, the key is to remain flexible and adapt the process to meet the cat's needs.

BEAMING REIKI:

Beaming Reiki is the process used when you are treating an unfamiliar or unfriendly cat. It can also be used to treat cats that are visible to you, but not immediately in front of you, such as cats being treated at an animal shelter.

Begin by asking permission from the cat to share Reiki energy with it. If the cat accepts the energy treatment, sit in a low chair or stool or on the ground and intend to provide Reiki energy for the cat. Extend your arms out with your palms facing outward (fingers pointing diagonally towards the ground/floor).

DISTANCE HEALING REIKI:

This method of treatment requires the Reiki Level II attunement in order to access the three Reiki practitioner symbols. These symbols create a stronger energy flow that permits deeper physical and emotional healing to take place. Sometimes a cat is much more receptive to energy sent to it from a distance than when it is offered in person; this is particularly true of cats that are dying.

The Reiki Power Symbol (abbreviated as CKR) increases the strength and flow of the Reiki energy. The Mental-Emotional Symbol (SHK) focuses deep healing on mental , emotional, and spiritual blockages that have manifested as physical or behavioral problems. The Distance-Healing Symbol HSZSN) helps you to send Reiki energy through time and space.

While Hands-on Reiki treatments can be anywhere from 15 – 60 minutes long, a Distance-Healing Reiki session usually lasts 15 – 30 minutes. Since you are not present in person with the cat when you do the treatment, you need to plan it for when the cat is normally inactive.

The Distance-Healing treatment process is as follows:

· Sit or stand in a relaxed manner.

· Draw the Distance-Healing Symbol in the air and say its mantra 3 times out loud.

· Place a picture of the cat in front of you and say its name (or a detailed description) 3 times out loud. Other options if a picture is not available are to:

Write the cat's name on a piece of paper, which is ten placed inside a small box. Reiki energy is then sent to the box at the appropriate time.

Use a stuffed bear as a treatment surrogate for the cat.

Use your own legs (when sitting down) to receive and to forward the Reiki energy to the cat. The following list identifies which of the cat's body parts correspond to parts of your legs:

1. The cat's head and neck (your left knee).

2. Heart and upper chest (your left mid-thigh).

3. Ribs and abdomen (your left upper thigh).

4. Pelvis (your left hip).

5. Back of head, neck, and throat (your right knee).

6. Shoulders and upper back (your right mid-thigh).

7. Mid and lower back (your right upper thigh).

8. Sacral area (your right hip).

· Draw the Mental-Emotional Symbol in the air and say its mantra 3 times out loud.

· Draw the Power Symbol in the air and say its mantra 3 times out loud.

- Then say, "With the help of the Reiki Symbols, I am now acting as a pure channel to send Reiki healing energy to (name of the cat. May this energy be only for the greatest and highest good of (name of the cat). So be it."

- Hold your hands with your palms facing outward, intend that Reiki flow to the cat for as long as you can sense energy flowing or for a pre-decided amount of time.

- NOTE on treatment frequency:

For animals recovering from an injury or illness, do a series of 3-4 treatments on consecutive days followed by once a week until recovery.

For healthy cats, once a week or as desired.

For cats nearing their transition, daily treatments or as desired.

- Concluding the Reiki treatment:

Cats will usually let you know when they have had enough energy by:

1. Waking up and moving away.

2. Becoming involved in another activity.

3. Licking your hands or touching you with their head.

You may terminate the session as well if you notice a significant decrease in the energy flowing through your hands.

Thank the cat and thank Reiki.

Chapter 8: Reiki Sessions: What To Expect

It is important to prepare yourself mentally, spiritually, and physically before a Reiki session. Setting your intention for your session will help you heal in the specific areas you need. Here is a step-by-step guide on preparing for a session.

Preparing for a Reiki session

Relax and reflect. Thirty minutes prior to your session, sit and meditate upon your emotions, mental state, and your physical sensations. What are you feeling? What jumps out at you the most? This is the time to set your intentions. It might be healing nausea and pain from cancer, joint pain from arthritis, or chronic migraines. Your issues might not be physical, but mental instead. Do you need to let go of anxiety from work? Depression from grief? Now is the time to focus on what is blocking your energy so you can help your practitioner focus on these issues too.

Relax and let go of all your stress and tension to help activate your own energy. Also, be sure to verbalize your needs to your healer before you begin your session.

EAT AND DRINK. A few hours before your session, eat a healthy, light meal and make sure you are adequately hydrated. Stick with non-caffeinated beverages like water, juice, or teas to stay away from caffeine which might make you jittery during your session. Nourishing and hydrating your body beforehand will allow you to focus on your energy and healing instead of hunger or thirst.

BE COMFORTABLE. Because you want to be in a completely relaxed state during your session, be sure to wear comfortable, stretchy clothing like yoga or stretch pants and a loose shirt. If you tend to get cold, bring socks and a light sweater or wrap to help keep you warm. Use the restroom before your session as well, since needing to go during a session may cause discomfort. Lastly, because you'll be lying down during your session, make sure to lie in a comfortable position and alert your practitioner if you are uncomfortable in any way.

The takeaway here is to prepare your body and mind before your session, taking care of essentials beforehand so you can completely focus on your healing without distractions.

Reiki Sessions for Beginners

Most people who have never had a Reiki session are very curious as to what a session entails. Learning what happens during a session beforehand might alleviate any anxiety or concerns you may have about the practice.

One aspect of Reiki healing is to find a trained practitioner to suit your needs. Take your time on this to find the right healer for you, and ask them how they structure their sessions. A typical Reiki session lasts one hour, although 90-minute sessions are available. You will be lying down fully reclined on a massage table. As stated previously, be sure to wear light, loose, comfortable clothing. Reiki is performed in two different ways. One way is with a light, gentle pressure static touch, or the no-hands method, where the practitioner's hands are a few centimeters or inches above your body. Let your healer know which method you prefer. Again, your comfort during a session is tantamount. For your first session, it is a good idea to arrive 10-15 minutes early to discuss your goals and needs and to complete any paperwork that might be needed.

During the Session

Most energy healing practitioners have their own dedicated space for sessions, but some make house calls. Healers usually play soft, calming music to help mask ambient noise, but let yours know if you prefer silence. You will lie down on a massage table (some patients need to be in chairs). The practitioner will then place or hover their hands over a series of locations on the head and front and back of the torso.

The feelings and sensations people feel during a session differ from person to person. Some people feel warmth from their healer's hands, while some experiencing a refreshing, cool touch. Others might feel subtle pulses from the practitioner's hands or cascading waves of pulsing sensations. The experience is subjective to each patient.

During the session, many people report falling asleep or falling into a deep, meditative sleep-like state. Some hover in a state of consciousness where they are aware of their surroundings while at the same time being deeply withdrawn. The most common sensation for most people is the feeling of relaxation and immediate release of tension and stress.

After the Session

Like with yoga, it is necessary and beneficial for you to take time to integrate your Reiki practice. After your session, keep your surroundings calm and quiet to extend your feelings of peace and tranquility. Some great ways to integrate your Reiki session would be to meditate and reflect on how you are feeling; take a walk outside in nature, especially in the woods or near water, as they are especially calming; or take a short nap. Try not to schedule any activities after a session, so you don't feel anxious about obligations.

It is also important to eat and drink after a session. Try to drink 1-2 glasses of water, and add electrolytes or drink a sports drink with electrolytes to replenish the body. Energy healing is work for the body, so you may also feel very hungry immediately after a session. Eat a light meal or healthy snack to ground the body and recenter the mind and spirit.

After you have replenished your body is a great time to reflect quietly on your practice. You can get creative during the reflection phase and write in a journal, draw, or paint to explore your sensations and emotions during your Reiki session. You can meditate to reflect in a quiet room, or you may prefer soft, calming music in the background.

If after your practice you feel any overwhelming emotions, mental distress, or physical pain, contact your practitioner for help and guidance. Even though Reiki is a gentle practice, the sudden free flow of energy may be overwhelming at first. Many people experience deep emotions after a Reiki session, which is completely normal and healthy. Just be sure to reach out to your practitioner if you feel you need assistance.

Chapter 9: basic Energy Anatomy

Anatomy doesn't mean just the different parts of your physical body. Anatomy is the study of the structures and the parts together, and just like your body has parts, so too does that part of you which is Energy.

As an introduction to energy anatomy, you will learn the concepts that have been mapped out and described by many cultures such as the double torus energy system, the aura fields, meridians, and chakras. To understand Reiki and energy healing, you need to first learn the concept of energy anatomy; what it is and how it works. Because this system is so diverse and beyond our own comprehension, it is important to understand that the pieces of it that we do know are just merely pieces. It has been my experience that most energy practitioners will notice different things. I believe the reason for this is because what we as individuals can see, feel, or know about the energy is transformed into something we can relate it to, so if someone is seeing colorful auric fields and someone else feels an energy blockage, who is right? Well they both are and they both have different ways of sensing and working with the energy. To make this even more complex and confusing one could even debate the fact that everyone is on different paths and whatever that person notices to work on is because it is something they are supposed to learn on their path as a healer, but for now we will focus on some basic knowledge that you can use to learn and grow from yourselves.

Double Torus

In this great age of scientific discoveries, we have now learned of the double torus energy flow. This energy is constantly swirling around us and cycling through, bringing in new energy and recycling old energy in figure 8 patterns around us. This swirling movement of energy body is found around everything no matter how big or how small, all the way down to the tiniest of molecules. The understanding of this energy system has led to a breakthrough in understanding how the energy is moved from outside our body and into our body. Not only does this energy flow surround our auric layer, but it is also connected to the constant flow of energy within our bodies, creating an influx of life energy into our system and pushing it through our energy fields.

Aura

All living things are surrounded by an energetic field, better known as an aura. It is believed that through this aura, we are all connected. It holds information about the object it surrounds by way of electromagnetic vibrations. This information can include the physical, emotional, mental, and spiritual map of the living thing it encompasses. In the case of our bodies, it is the very energy of life. All living beings create energy. Our heart's rhythm creates an electric pulse which can be monitored by sensitive equipment. We create our own individual magnetic fields, and we even have polarized sides (positive and negative) the basis for polarity therapy, another energy healing modality. The mystics of the world learned to characterize and use this energy. They realized sometimes too much energy was lost and an imbalance was created, which in turn caused sickness. The 3 main layers you will work with are:

***1. Physical Body*-** This layer extends out about an inch or two from the body. It is most often the easiest layer to see and sense. This layer of energy reflects the bones, muscles, and organs, and also includes the first layer of the energy body, sometimes called the "etheric template". It is within this layer Shamanic practitioners can scan the body to find sources of injury, pain and disease.

2. Mental/Emotional Body – This is the next layer that extends out a few feet from the body. This is what most people see as the colored portion of the auric body that forms a bubble around the individual. This layer holds mental and emotional processes and reactions, as well as long-term standing patterns as the emotional/mental reflections of diseases. This layer has many more layers within it, each with a different meaning and connection.

3. *Divine Self-* The final layer is connected to the Higher Self and with the Divine. It is not limited to the personality, gender, or history we carry around with us in a given lifetime; instead it is the spiritual body of who we really are as it reaches out from our soul. It rises so high above us that it connects us to all living things and it extends infinitely. It is in this layer we can

find out more about who someone really is.

Meridians

The Chinese system of meridians dates back to the beginning of their recorded medical practices. The meridians are energy pathways through the body that connect the energy to the various organ systems. These lines have many points on them which are believed to stimulate organ function. Blockages or stagnant energy in the meridian lines cause dysfunction and disease within the physical body. This energy theory is the basis for acupressure and acupuncture treatments, as well as reflexology. In Reiki we do not work specifically with the meridians however we do affect their function, so it is important to understand how these systems work together. All of these systems come from different cultures and beliefs, yet they are all correct pieces of the puzzle that make up our energy body.

Ayurvedic Chakras

Ayurvedic energy theory defines three major pathways: the central channel; the masculine polarity channel; and the feminine polarity channel. The feminine channel receives charged prana (energy) through the left nostril; the masculine channel receives charged prana through the right nostril. This energy circulates in the body and goes through the central and most important channel down through the body and filters into the various energy centers (chakras). There are seven major chakras located along the **central channel**. Each contains life-energy vibrating at a specific level. They correspond to various vital functions, emotional states, physical organs and even senses. The seven main chakras include: Root, Sacrum, Solar Plexus, Heart, Throat, Third Eye, and Crown.

How the energy fields work together

Our aura is the energy layer which allows us to feel connected to everything, protects us, warns us, picks up on other energies and surrounds everything. The energies we come in contact with leave energetic markings in our auric field. If we come in contact with a negative person we may feel that negative energy within seconds or within hours depending on how our energy system is flowing within the double torus pattern. The auric layer passes some energy onto the chakra system. The chakra centers draw in this energy as it is pushed through our aura by the double torus movement. This energy comes in through our crown and flows down to the other chakras as the double torus movement continues to push the energy around our body, causing each chakra vortex to spin. As this flow gets to our root chakra it is filtered again as it is sent out to the earth through our root and feet, then the recycled earthy energy is sent back up. Now this cycled energy gets sent through the meridian system as it travels up the legs and feet and meets at the root, it then branches off through these energetic veins and arteries (the meridian lines) and flows to our organs, muscle tissue, blood, lymph, and glandular system. This is how energy is able to affect our physical bodies. There is much more depth to how our energy system works, as there are MANY more energy pathways than this, but this will provide you with a great start to build some understanding of these complex energy systems.

Shamanic Energy Work

In Shamanic healing, practitioners work on energetic dysfunctions by removing blockages, clearing energy pathways, increasing energy, and ensuring proper flow of energy. Some people see energy, others feel it, and some just know. The way you connect to the energy is not as important as being open to receive and interpret the information. Once you have become skilled at working in the energy field, it becomes easier to access the different realms where energy is constantly moving, changing, and shifting. It is within these deeper layers of existence that Shamanic practitioners work. There are many exercises you can do to help build your intuition when working with energy, but ultimately it relies on your ability to connect and receive information through energy.

Shamanic healing encompasses a wide range of energy work modalities. What makes Shamanic work different is that it also incorporates the use of spiritual allies, whether it be angels, guides, ascended masters, the Divine, animals, or plants. The spiritual energetic essences of these beings are called in to aid in the healing process. It can be as easy as saying a prayer before session asking for their aid, or as complex as using animal totem spirits to help with a specific problem the client faces. It is through this spiritual connection we learn to live in harmony within our physical realm and the realm of energy.

Energy Practice

If you have ever experienced *knowing* that someone was staring at you without seeing them, or you have *felt* someone walk up behind you although you had no way of knowing they did, then you have sensed it through your auric body. It is often referred to as a "sense" or an "intuition". The first step in learning about your aura is learning to feel it.

Practice exercise 1: Work with a partner. One person sits with their eyes closed and arms held out. The other person will then begin by holding their hand 12 inches above the seated persons arm. Slowly you will lower your hand towards the arm (pick one of their arms). As you lower your hands, the seated person will let you know when they feel you. This exercise will show you how far out you are able to "feel" your aura. Once you have completed the exercise, switch positions and repeat.

Practice exercise 2: Start in a dimly lit room and in a relaxed and comfortable position. Now squeeze your hands together, palm to palm for about 2 minutes. Then drop your hands by your sides. Now slowly raise your hands, palms facing, bringing your hands closer together until you feel a magnetic pull between them. Don't let the palms touch. To take this exercise to the next level, adjust your gaze to be slightly off focus from the center of your hands. You may be able to see the halo of color, or aura, around them. It is often felt as a tingling or pulsating feeling.

How did the energy feel to you? What did you see?

Chapter 10: How To Practice Reiki On Yourself

Techniques for Practicing Reiki on Yourself

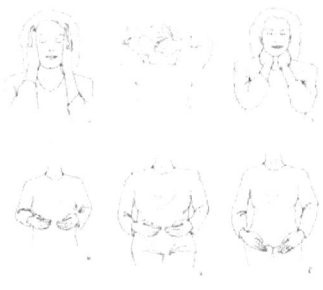

Like the beginning of Reiki in level one, the focus on clearing your mind, body, and soul effectively, which is essential for self-practice.

Once you have achieved this successfully, you'll be able to prepare yourself for Reiki self-treatment, and this can be done with regularity (this is recommended), as it will enhance the quality of your life and those around you.

To prepare for Reiki, consider taking the following steps:

●Recognize Reiki's universal power and its accessibility.

It is not a separate entity that we gain access to, but rather, it exists in all of us, and we can connect with it at any time through channels.

●Your body has the natural ability to heal itself, and Reiki is a means to support and strengthen this process.

●It's important to feel a sense of peace and comfort during Reiki treatment.

This will support the outcome of each session. If you feel upset or agitated, a few minutes of self-guided meditation can help.

This will allow you to clear the negative energy away in preparation for treatment.

- Find a quiet space where you can comfortably begin treatment on yourself.

This may be a private location at home or in a quiet office when you are alone and without interruption.

It is important to be alone, so you can solely focus on your own needs and healing.

If you require assistance during a healing session, consult with someone who is experienced with Reiki, or another person that you trust to observe and help you if needed.

- Consider starting your sessions by yourself with no music or background noise at all.

This may be difficult if you live in an urban area or often surrounded by noise (even if minimal).

Try your best to find a quiet and distraction-free area, and if this means taking a trip outside to a beach or quiet forest, this may work as well.

When you're ready to begin, you'll need to prepare the space where you wish to practice Reiki on yourself.

It is recommended that the same, comfortable place be used for each session unless you need to move for reasons outside of your control.

Eventually, once you have completed a few treatments, you may want to add some soft, background music or calming sounds, such as ocean waves or a running brook.

The following elements will help improve your self-practice experience:

● Use pillows, blankets, and other soft props to give yourself a cozy space to relax during treatment. These can be kept regularly in the same space for convenience and ease of use.

● Treat yourself regularly, even daily, if you can.

The more often the treatment, the greater the benefit you'll experience.

If you find that the quietest or calm period of time is in the early morning or late into the evening, for example, use one of these time frames to schedule your self-treatment session.

●Sometimes you may not feel well or energetic enough to complete a session.

If you can and are able to, it's best to proceed, even if it means a shorter time or less intense treatment.

The reason for continuing through any state of being, whether you feel well or not, is because Reiki will especially benefit you if you're feeling sick and lacking energy.

In fact, this is the ideal time to focus on treatment and continue with regularity.

●Time frames are flexible and can work within a tight schedule if this is a dilemma.

Just twenty minutes a day can make a significant difference.

This can be done twice a day, or for longer sessions, once a day, for 45-60 minutes.

Choose a plan, including a time span and frequency that works within your lifestyle, while making your health and space for treatment a priority as well.

•Choose a position that works best for you in your space.

This may be lying down, sitting, or leaning back on a reclining chair, for example.

You may want to try a few positions until you find one most suitable.

Create a situation that works best for increasing your ability to relax and receive the treatment.

Before you begin, remember that Reiki self-practice is important for you.

It's vital for your well-being, and you deserve to feel its benefit for self-improvement and wellness.

Proceeding with a session begins with making yourself comfortable by using the tips and suggestions outlined above.

Keep it simple at first and ensure that your space of choosing does not contain any distractions.

Put aside your technology, books and other items that can easily sway our attention.

When you are ready for your first session of self-practice, implement the following steps:

Remove your shoes, dim the lights (if this helps you relax), and make yourself comfortable in your chosen space.

Make sure there is no background noise or sounds that can distract you. If there is noise outside, close the window, and if there is a television or radio playing in the background or in another room, turn it down or off completely.

Recline or prepare yourself in your most comfortable position. If desired, prop your knees with a pillow to allow for better circulation in the body.

Close your eyes and take a mental note of the purpose of the session. This is your time and space to heal and be comfortable.

Breathe evenly and slowly, creating calm within, and prepare to place your hands in the areas of your body that you need or wish to focus on. Continue for as long as you can or until you are satisfied with the results.

If you live with others, let them know when and where you will be self-practicing, so they are aware and can accommodate as best as possible.

Choose a regular time of day to practice Reiki, to avoid conflict with your schedule and others in your household. Keeping a regular time allows you to anticipate the treatment, and looking forward to it every day.

The Benefits of Self-Practice

The ability and power to be able to heal yourself and benefit from the power of Reiki are amazing, and why self-practice is a great way to improve your life.

There are many benefits associated with self-practice, especially when it is done regularly as an important part of your life.

While the treatment is simple in practice, it can result in some powerful effects that greatly improve the quality of your life:

●The reduction of stress is one of the top reasons for self-practicing Reiki.

It allows your mind and focus to drift away from items or situations in life that cause us stress and build tension in our bodies. We often do not realize how harmful stress can be until it becomes debilitating and affects other parts of our well-being.

For this reason, Reiki is powerful in that it strips away the stressors, allowing our minds to freely float away from tension and find true peace.

- A better sense of harmony and peace can be achieved through self-treatment.

This includes slowing down any anger or frustration we may hold onto because of an uncontrollable situation at work or a family disagreement.

These treatment sessions allow us to focus solely on the peace and harmony aspect of life and how important this is for our health.

- You'll be able to let go of fear and the stress factors that are attached to it.

During a session of Reiki, you have the ability to harness incredible energy that will give you the strength to handle situations that cause fear and intimidation, by approaching them with a renewed sense of peace and a goal of resolving situations, rather than allowing them to fester and cause us grief.

- Our bodies can self-heal through a process called parasympathetic or through the nervous system.

This ability is heightened or increased during a session of self-treatment.

The benefits of self-healing include a better quality of rest or sleep at night, with fewer chances of interruption or distraction, as well as improved digestion and immune system function.

- Reiki will enhance the success of other treatments you may take or need for various medical and health conditions.

For example, if a specific medication creates side effects, or the idea of experiencing side effects from certain medical treatments causes worry or anticipation of the negative experience, Reiki can diffuse this sensation of worry and allow you to become calmer, more receptive to the therapy/therapies while enjoying the relaxation of self-practice.

●If you have sustained physical injury from an accident or are in the process of recovering from surgery, Reiki is non-invasive, as it doesn't require much touch (if any), and it is gentle.

This is a major benefit when practicing on yourself and others. Reiki becomes a bridge between experiencing the discomfort of injury towards recovery and healing, without being invasive or risking further damage.

●Many people experience a spiritual benefit with Reiki, in how it helps them improve their spiritual growth and strive for personal improvement.

While some people may not consider themselves spiritual or religious at all, they may still feel a sense of deep satisfaction and inner peace with self-practice.

Some people report feeling a better sense of being able to make better decisions in life that have a greater, more positive impact on them and others' lives around them.

This form of guidance, as some may consider it, can lead people to make incredible changes in their lives that benefit them significantly, such as quitting smoking, getting more involved in the family, and improving the relationship with people.

- You only need level one for self-practice.

In fact, many people take this level (at the beginner stage), so they can use the new methods of energy channeling to benefit themselves.

The benefits of self-practice, over time, often encourage people to continue their studies further, so they can increase the energy levels through attunements and make the best of Reiki treatment.

Chapter 11: Benefits Of Crystal For Reiki

Reiki as a standalone modality is extremely effective even without the use of crystals. It is likely though that you have been drawn to Crystal Reiki because you are ready to add the unique energy it provides to your work. Performing Crystal Reiki sessions can help you to focus on specific conditions that clients are eager to have addressed. Not all of your Reiki sessions have to include crystals and you may find when working with a client initially that you choose to perform traditional Reiki sessions.

As the client's healing progresses, you and they may want to hone in one of the specific issues they are concerned with. Crystal Reiki can provide that focus.

In other cases you may find that a single condition is so pervasive in the client's overall sense of wellbeing that it needs to be addressed first before balancing on a widespread level can occur. In these cases you can begin with Crystal Reiki sessions and then use traditional sessions as you feel called to.

Clients who are not in tune with their energy or the frequencies around them may have a difficult time perceiving energy in a traditional Reiki session. Crystals are tangible forms of energy. Although they are beautiful objects that we can hold, they also hold powerful energetic vibrations that can be sensed.

Using crystals can help clients tune into the energetic level which in turn can reassure them that shifts are happening. This reassurance is what helps them to make the conscious choice to return for more sessions and healing. Although in your traditional Reiki sessions you are using your intuition to guide you as you move from position to position and receive information from the recipient's bodymind, in Crystal Reiki your playground has more for you to explore.

You will use your intuition to help you choose the crystals as well as the special layout they will be placed in. During the session you can tune into each crystal for information it may have as well as the combined energies of the crystals as Reiki flows through them. In your traditional Reiki sessions, you likely included grounding techniques for yourself and your recipient at the end and/or beginning of your sessions.

Crystals naturally provide that energy so your sessions will be infused with the higher frequency energy of Reiki as well as the centering energy of the earth. You may also find working with crystals in your distance Reiki practice very helpful. In place of performing a traditional Reiki distance session, you can create a crystal grid connected to the recipient and their needs and allow it to draw in Reiki energy each day.With the foundation of Traditional Reiki with you, you can use

Crystal Reiki to take your practice to exciting and wondrous new levels.

The 3 Pillars of Modern Reiki

The three pillars of modern reiki are a great example of a ritual that enhances the reiki session. It allows the practitioner to connect with their higher self along with the reiki source. This formula is broken up into three parts which are; gassho, reji-ho and chiryo.

Within these three pillars are their own individual attributes. When synchronized together, as with any ritual, we gain a deeper connection to that intent.

Reiki is a Japanese healing technique based on the principle that the practitioner channels energy into the patient by means of touch to activate the natural healing processes of the patient's body. The word reiki is made up of two Japanese words: rei meaning "God's wisdom" or "the higher power" and ki which means "life force energy." Reiki restores physical and emotional well-being in a manner that is relaxing and nonevasive to the client.

The First Pillar: Gassho

The first pillar of Reiki, gassho, is more than a meditative practice. It also serves as a form of spiritual hygiene, a ritual to create intention and focus, an invitation to mindfulness, a call to set aside ego, and the primary method to invite and ignite Reiki healing energy within a session.

While gassho is primarily taught in modern forms of Reiki as a meditative practice that entails holding one's hands in prayer position and focusing on where the middle fingertips meet, it is far more involved and deeper than these simple instructions indicate.

During gassho, while the fingertips serve as a physical focal point to help the Reiki practitioner remain mindful and in the moment, a skilled practitioner combines the mindfulness of gassho with breath work and intention.

As spiritual hygiene: As spiritual hygiene, Reiki practitioners should engage in gassho for 5 to 10 minutes before every session in order to purify not only the energy of the space in which the sacred sharing of the Reiki energy will occur, but also to enter into a state of mindfulness where he or she is open to Reiki energy and positive guidance. This is especially important for practitioners who live "normal" lives between sessions (and don't we all?) where the needs of the world often intrude on upon our ideal spiritual state of being.

Before every session, perform any energy work in your healing space you normally do as part of your pre-game ritual, whether that involves burning herbs, drawing symbols in the space, or any other space clearing ritual. Next, sit comfortably in the space in gassho.

Concentrate on your breathing and the space where your middle fingertips meet. Feel Reiki forming in the air around you and breathe it in, allowing it to flow in through your nose and lungs and throughout your entire body.

Exhale tension or anything from your day that does serve you nor not belong in your session. Do this for as long as it takes. Some days, it may only take five minutes, but on those other days where the world has intruded, it may take longer. Do this until you are calm, peaceful, centered, and out of your ego.

Only then should you invite your healing partner into your healing space.

To Set Intention, Invite and Ignite Reiki Energy: Once you have invited your healing partner into the appropriately prepared space, consulted with them as needed, and they are resting comfortably on your treatment table, stand at your partner's head or feet and enter into gassho again. This time, do so focusing on any intention for the session you and your healing partner have agreed upon along with the intention to serve the highest and greatest good. Once again, feel the Reiki gather around you. Breathe it in, and invite it to flow through you and into your hands. When you feel your hands ignite, you can begin your session.

To Return to Mindfulness or Seek Guidance: Throughout your session, you can return to gassho any time you feel the need. Gassho is your safe space where you can return to mindfulness, refocus or reset intention, or receive guidance about where to place your hands on your healing partner. It is the form within the freedom of an intuitive Reiki session. If you feel your mind start to drift or notice your energy shift, return to gassho. If you feel unsure about what to do next, return to gassho. Walk to your partner's head or feet again and stand in gassho until you feel refocused. If you need, ask for guidance and then pay attention. A thought may come into your head, a part of your healing partner's body may "light up" in your gaze, or you may just feel drawn to a certain area. Go with this flow. Return to gassho whenever you need to recenter, wish to return to mindfulness if the outside world starts to intrude on your session, or feel unsure of what to do next.

To Give Thanks and Return to Yourself: You can also return to gassho at the close of a session. When you feel ready, move to your healing partner's feet and stand in gassho. Give thanks to Reiki and to your partner for allowing you to channel the energy to serve the highest and greatest good. Then, invite your energy to return to you and see the energetic connection between you and your partner releasing. When you feel ready, run your hands under cool water or touch the ground to ground yourself.

The Second Pillar: Reiji-Ho

Gassho is interwoven throughout the other two pillars of Reiki. Reiji-ho, the second pillar, is all about asking for guidance. While First Degree Reiki practitioners learn the Reiki hand positions, as they progress they may begin to feel comfortable enough to work intuitively. I encourage students entering Second Degree Reiki to begin working intuitively as often as possible during Reiki sessions knowing if they need to, they can always return to the hand positions.

In reiji-ho, you invite guidance in. It begins in gassho, with your hands held in prayer position asking to have your hands and energy guided to serve the highest and greatest good of your healing partner. And then, you wait and you use all of your senses to listen.

Listen to how your body feels, what your mind thinks, what your eyes see, and how your healing partner responds. As you wait for guidance, observe with all of your senses and allow your mind to empty so it becomes a vessel into which guidance can flow easily.

You will learn over time how your Divine Guidance signals you. You may spot a twitch. You may feel something in your own body. You may hear instructions in your mind. You may feel as if you are magnetically drawn to somewhere on your healing partner's body. There is no wrong way to receive information.

Reiji-ho takes trust in yourself, your healing partner, your Divine Guidance system, Reiki, and the universe. It also requires mindfulness. It requires you to allow yourself to be energetically open in order to become a vessel the universe uses to serve the highest and greatest good. When you receive a signal, trust it, act on it, and know the Reiki energy will flow exactly where and as it is needed for the highest and greatest good.

When you feel yourself slipping out of that space as a vessel and a channel and back into your own personal stuff, return to gassho and re-set yourself.

Third Pillar: Chiryo

The third pillar of Reiki, chiryo, is all about action.

Chiryo means "treatment," and it is an essential part of every Reiki session. New Reiki practitioners focus primarily on chiryo, following the mechanical process of placing hands on the body in set positions and trusting the Reiki will flow where it's needed.

However, as a practitioner becomes more deeply involved in the true practice of Reiki, chiryo is something that flows and changes depending on intuitive information the Reiki practitioner receives and the needs of his or her healing partner.

A practitioner truly engaged in chiryo moves beyond the basic hand positions and sometimes even moves beyond use of the hands. He or she may be intuitively guided to gaze, tap, stroke, blow, or visualize along with placing hands, palms, or fingertips in the ways they are guided to do so. In this way, a mindful session of

Reiki becomes a flowing dance of energy that involves the practitioner, his or her healing partner, and the entire universe.

How to start Practising Reiki

Not everyone who practices Reiki wants to use their training as a means to make a living. However, serving as a healer can be a very satisfying career. As a Reiki practitioner, you can take pride in your work and make a difference in your clients' quality of life.If you are thinking about setting up a Reiki practice, consider the following tips before getting started.

➢ GET CERTIFIED: There are three levels of basic training in Usui Reiki. You only need to be certified in the first level of training to offer Reiki treatments to clients. You will need to be certified in all levels in order to teach classes and give Reiki attunements to students.

➢ BECOME COMFORTABLE GIVING REIKI TREATMENTS: It is best not to jump in feet first setting up a Reiki practice until you have a clear understanding of your relationship with the workings of Reiki. Begin experiencing Reiki on a personal level through self-treatments and treating family members and friends. Experiencing all the inner workings of this gentle, complex healing art takes time. Reiki clears away blockages and imbalances gradually. Allow Reiki to help you get your own life in balance before taking on the task of helping others.

➢ CHOOSE A WORK LOCATION: Reiki sessions are being offered in hospitals, nursing homes, pain management clinics, spas, and home-based businesses. The benefit of working in a hospital, clinic, spa, or elsewhere is that appointment bookings and insurance claim filings are usually taken care of for you. Most health insurances do not reimburse for Reiki treatments, but a few do. Medicare sometimes pays for Reiki treatments if the sessions are prescribed for pain management. Practicing from a home-based office is a dream come true for many practitioners, but this convenience comes with issues to consider. Do you have a room or area within your home, separate from your normal living quarters, that could be dedicated to healing? Does the residential zone you are living in allow home-based businesses? And, there is also the safety issue of inviting strangers into your personal living space to consider.

➢ GATHER YOUR EQUIPMENT AND SUPPLIES: You will want to invest in a sturdy massage table for your practice if the space you'll be practicing in doesn't have one. If you offer to travel in order to make home visits or give treatments in hotel rooms, a portable massage table will be necessary. Here is a checklist of equipment and supplies for your Reiki practice:

Massage table

Table accessories (face rest, bolster, carrying case, etc)

Swivel chair with rollers

Freshly cleaned linens

Blankets

Pillows

Tissues

Bottled water

➢ ADVERTISE YOUR REIKI PRACTICE: Word of mouth is a good way to get started working as a Reiki practitioner. Let your friends and relatives know that you're open for business. Have business cards printed up and distribute them freely at local bulletin boards at libraries, community colleges, natural food markets, etc. Offer introductory workshops and Reiki shares to educate your community about Reiki.

In the modern era, word of mouth also means having a presence on social media. Setting up a Facebook page for your practice is free and only takes a few minutes. Ideally, you'll have your own website that lists your location and contact information, but if that's out of reach, a Facebook page is a good start to draw in new clients. Facebook also has tools that allow small businesses to reach a targeted audience (costs will vary).

➢ SET YOUR REIKI FEES: Research what other Reiki practitioners are charging in your area for their services. You will want to be competitive, but don't undercut yourself. Do a cost-benefit analysis and know how much you need to earn—whether it's per hour, per patient or per treatment—to cover your expenses and have some money left over. If you arrange to treat clients outside of your home, chances are you will either pay a fixed rate for a rental space or share a percentage of your session fees with your host business. Keep good records of the money you are earning. Working as an independent contractor involves being informed of your income tax and self-employment obligations.

➢ OFFER FREE REIKI EVENINGS: A free Reiki evening can create lots of interest. Plan one night a month to talk about Reiki and give sample treatments. If you have Reiki friends, ask them to come and help give treatments. This is a great way to help others and let them know about Reiki and your practice. Make up flyers for your free Reiki evening and put them up in appropriate places. If the Reiki practitioners can meet an hour or so before the meeting to give treatments to each other it will really improve the quality of what the non-Reiki people receive. Also, if you have taken Reiki III/master training, you could give a refresher attunement or healing attunement to each of the practitioners to boost their energy. This is a great way for the practitioners to practice their Reiki and for you to practice giving attunements. Call everyone you know who would be interested and let them know.If your area has psychic or wholistic fairs, get a booth. Take a Reiki table and ask 5 or more of your Reiki friends to help. Offer 10 or 15 minute treatments with 5 or more Reiki practitioners giving a treatment to one person at a time. Charge $10.00 or so per treatment. This can be a powerful healing experience and a good demonstration of Reiki. Have a table with your flyers and business cards on it and be sure to get each persons name, address, and phone number for your mailing list. Another way is to use chairs and have one or two practitioners give 10 or 15 minutes for each person.

Chapter 12: Sun Ancon Chi Machine

I love how we have so many ways to help ourselves and the right person comes into our lives at the right time. The Chi machine was invented by a doctor of oxygen in Japan. He wanted to help people get more oxygen into their bodies without them having to exercise. He saw Koi Carp swimming in a figure of eight and soon after helped a person by swinging her legs in the same way. After this, he went on to invent the first Chi machine. It is now used worldwide and in hospitals too. I remember being told of a patient's group in a hospital buying one for the staff to use during their breaks. Another eye surgeon let his patients use the machine before they were operated on. The chi machine both gives more energy to people and helps them relax. They also found during trials that it removed excess fluid from the body which was very helpful for people suffering from Lymphoedema. What's not to like in this machine?

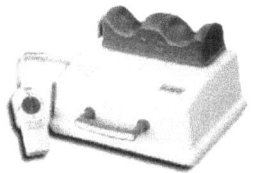

The person that introduced me to the chi machine probably does not know how much of an impact this made on my life. He advised me that he had suffered from Cancer and that had caused him to have back problems, so it may help me too and he was right. This also came about synchronically. I met him through my social group on a holiday. He was from England and without the group I would never have met him or heard about this machine. I decided to do a lot more research on the Sun Ancon Chi machine. I found it was the original one and many years had gone into research before making it, so I was completely comfortable about spreading the word and decided to become a distributor of it.

This machine can help many health issues as it gives you a gentle massage and a boost of energy at the end. The most important point for me is it was also a form of exercise that would not put my back out. Once I started using it, I wanted to shout from the rooftops the response my body was getting from it. After eight weeks I had forgotten I had a bad back.

When my daughter was married a few months later I had danced the twist with my other two-year-old grandson. Of course, my back did not like this and went into crisis mode again.

The most unfortunate thing was my Osteopath was on holiday and the two osteopaths that I saw told me not to use my chi machine and to apply cold to my back. As before I had always given myself warm baths and used my chi machine, I should not have been surprised that my back did not improve. When my own practitioner returned the damage was done and it took seven weeks for my back to recover. Before this I had only needed one or two days away from my workplace. He advised me I should have done what I normally did and to stick to this in the future. The people I had seen while he was away had treated me for a new injury when it was referred pain from my existing problems. The good thing was my work was very accommodating and allowed me to take my chi machine into work so that every hour or two I could relax the muscles in my back which allowed me to stay in the office. Since that day I have seen him only a couple of times, just to check all is okay if my back goes, and he always tells me just to keep using the chi machine.

One day I had a therapy event to go with my chi machines and thought how could I do this? My back had gone while I was putting a bottle of water into a bag. How could I even drive to the place? I did not think I would be able to sit in a car, never mind drive. I used the Sun Ancon Chi machine in my home and then got someone to take it out to the car. I was then able to drive forty minutes. As soon as I got to the destination, I had this person set up my exercise mat and machine and went straight back on it again. After ten minutes I was able to stand all day till 4.30pm before I started having problems again. This machine is a miracle worker for me.

You can see what was happening here. All the things that helped me with my health were to do with energy. The crystals, reiki and the Sun Ancon Chi machine were giving me tools not only to help myself but others too. I often find now that clients like to use reiki and crystals at the same time and then they finish off with some time on the Sun Ancon Chi Machine.

After I had recovered, I wanted to make more people aware of the chi machine and started taking it into the therapy shop with me at the weekends. It helps people to relax and chill out, so they did not need to have any health issues. One memory I have is when we were having a weekend of taster sessions. One lady advised me she had many mental health problems. After speaking to her and realising that the issues were severe, and she had not been attending her clinic, I advised that I could not give 15 minutes of reiki as I thought she may become emotional and need a lot more time which I did not have on that day. I suggested she use the chi machine instead.

After a few minutes she was lying very relaxed and asked me if the machine would work with the drug Speed. I asked her why and was astounded by her answer. She had taken some just before she entered the therapy shop! I asked her how she was feeling, and she advised very chilled out, so I told her she had the answer - not that I would recommend this to anyone. She also asked that I told her husband in the car waiting on her that she was too relaxed to move. I often find after using the machine that people are so relaxed, they just want to stay on the floor, but this took it to a new limit!

I have since found that the Sun Ancon chi machine is great for people who are stressed or have mental health issues. One of my friends had a highly stressful job and could not switch off at night. When she tried the machine, she said her head felt empty for the first time in years. I have frequently been told by clients that it clears their minds and I can attest to this too. I have found also it helps people with MS, ME and Fibromyalgia. It is unfortunate at this time that more and more people are being diagnosed with the latter two. I think we are living in a sick world now with the amount of pollution and chemicals we put into our bodies daily. This is bound to be influencing our bodies. Also, more and more people are being found to have mental health issues and depression. I think many people struggle to live with the high levels of stress they or circumstances put upon them these days too.

I was lucky to be able to take the chi machines into my work with a national company during their Health and Wellbeing days and it was great to see people getting chilled out within minutes. I remember one lady tell me her baby had finally gone to sleep while she was lying on the floor. It had been very restless up till that point. I told her my daughter went through a period in her pregnancy that the baby kept waking her in the middle of the night. She found if she got out of the bed and went on the chi machine for a few minutes the baby went back to sleep. As she also had pelvic dysplasia, she found it helped immensely with this as well.

I especially remember a day at work when we were in a room that if there was no movement, the energy efficient lights would go off. I had three people lying on the floor and switched on all their machines. Within a couple of minutes, the lights switched off. When the machines finally switched off the clients lay still as I had advised. The atmosphere was so peaceful, and everyone was relaxed until one of them moved and the lights all switched back on again. All I heard then was "bright lights, bright lights!" It was quite funny.

Usually when I took the chi machines into the office, I would have all my colleagues standing watching those using the machines as it looks quite funny when you see people's bodies moving in a figure of eight. They would then goad all their friends to take a session on the chi machines. Feedback was always good; in fact, one person said to me that if they had a call with a member of the public that upset them then a few minutes on this machine would clear their heads and calm them down. Perhaps a Sun Ancon chi machine should be in every workplace. If you want to check it out information can be found on my website here:

I now found myself with multiple therapies under my belt which I had never anticipated. This was all self-development for me, but I loved the fact I was now able to share all three with members of the public. My reiki, crystals and chi machine were now able to help so many people as they also helped me. I found friends and family would pay me extra visits to use them. I got to know many people's stories and had them all leaving with smiles on their faces. Life was good, and I loved it.

I remember taking a couple to a Body and Soul fair in Edinburgh. One of the stall holders kept coming across to where I had people lying on the floor. During a break he advised me that I should have a video playing above. When I asked him why he said that every time the machine switched off, he had to race across to see the look on people's faces! When the machines stop, people get a burst of energy going up their body.

I always remember a person that was in my house trying one out. He said, "Who needs drugs when you can feel like that!" I looked at him as he quickly added "Of course I don't do drugs." I even had a client visit me with her husband. She said to me "Tell him what time you go to bed and how many hours you sleep". I told him 12am till 6am and that I had to force myself to bed, knowing I had work a few hours later. She then said that she had advised her husband that she had never seen someone with so much energy!

Master/ Teacher Training

The thing about reiki is it has a mind of its own. I say it chose me and sends me in the direction it wants me to go. After a time, I kept getting a feeling more was to happen. It was like someone kept knocking at my door. I discussed this with my reiki teacher, and he asked me if I would like to go to the next level. I said I was not sure as it was too much money and I could never afford this. Also, I thought I would have no use for the next level. He suggested we put a date in the diary, for almost a year away, and if it was meant to happen, I would have the money before the date. I agreed to this while at the back of my mind thinking it would not happen due to lack of money, so unlike the earlier reiki training, I was not building my hopes up. Also, I thought the next level of training was only for training others. How wrong I was, and synchronicity kicked in again.

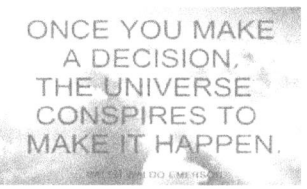

By this time, I had become a distributor for the Sun Ancon Chi machine to spread the word and had already sold a couple, so I put the commission money into an account to add to what I had already saved. I then got money for Christmas again but was about £39 short of the full amount that I needed for the workshop and had no idea where this would come from. Now this may not seem a lot of money to you but back then it was for me. I then got the worst bonus from work that I had ever had. You guessed it- £39. I was on my way. This was my way of knowing that I was taking the right direction in my life. I always said that if you went to the next level that you would make reiki your life and I was not wrong.

The time arrived for my long weekend of training and I went with my teacher David to a lovely cottage in a very quiet village in Scotland for one to one training. While we were on our way, he asked me why was I doing this training? Was it to make money? I advised that I felt it was something I needed to do for me and my family. He was pleased that I did not want to use it in a monetary way. He asked if I would want to train people in reiki and then I uttered words I will never forget. I said I had promised to train my daughter only and no one else. After laughing his words were "Watch this space". I should have taken notice. Once again, my life was about to change but always for the better.

There were only another two or three cottages close by and in front of us was the sea. When I looked out into the back garden, I could see partridges wandering around. It was so peaceful and the most perfect place to learn my Usui Master and Teacher qualifications. It made such an impact on me that later I decided this was the way for me to teach also. I would also always work with very small groups or individuals. This has stayed with me and I feel that I have made lots of friends from many of the people I have trained. I believe this is down to giving personal attention rather than being one of a large group.

I have been blessed to have the same teacher for all my levels and learned so much from him. One thing I took from my training was to make sure people knew they could come back to me if they needed any more information as they grew with the energy. If I did not have the answer, I would pass the question to David and would always get the information I needed. I also learned that at each level there is so much for the mind to take in that it is good to have a period between each level. Reiki is a wonderful gift to be added to your life

and it should be enjoyed rather than rushed through. It has been shown to me many times that everyone adjusts to the energy differently and some need more time than others between each level. It is for this reason, I do not believe in giving level one and two together.

During the weekend things went at a very easy pace and when we wanted, we would take a walk or give each other reiki. I cannot put into words the effect this time had on me. Up until that weekend I always said I struggled meditating. As part of the weekend, I was asked to do some meditations. During one meditation a very special bird came to me. Since then I have had it on all my business information. People often now call me the Swan lady. I remember after the weekend was over David sent me a link to T Rex's song Ride a White Swan! I certainly felt after that weekend I was flying high.

It often surprises me that people rush through reiki and take part in websites that offer training all over distance. In these days of wanting bargains I always think you get what you pay for. Experience and practise as one to one, for me, wins hands over all the time. I have been shocked to see some distance training being done with no space in between the levels. To say you can become a Reiki Master / Teacher in a weekend really worries me as people than then go out in the public and charge to both give reiki and attune others. Therefore, the UK Reiki

Federation will only register you if you have trained in person. I can understand people wanting to learn to heal themselves as reiki is a fantastic modality but before you go and teach, I strongly believe you need a lot more interaction and practice. How can this be done with no one checking on how you are working? When I think of the students I have trained over the years, some have needed more practice and guidance than others to feel secure in the knowledge that they are doing the right thing. Another thing about distance and especially all the cheap deals out there is that some people may have no back up if they have questions after being trained. These may arise months or even years after training so it's always good to check with any teacher about this before paying out any money.

Another thing you should ask of anyone training you in reiki is to see their Lineage. This shows who trained them, going all the way back to Dr Usui.

Chapter 13: Health Improvement

Stress and Relaxation

The most obvious, instantaneous, and dramatic benefit of Reiki is its ability to decrease stress and increase relaxation. This is because Reiki was actually discovered and designed for the express purpose of turning on your body's switch for relaxation. The reason it is so effective at doing so is because your body naturally wants to heal itself, and so using Reiki activates that skill inside of yourself.

In today's technologically advanced, always connected, constantly trying to be more efficient, more effective, and more productive than ever world that we live in, the number of manifestations that stress takes on the body is astronomical. So for most people, this simple benefit is the most life-changing and rewarding aspect of performing Reiki. Be helping to eliminate the negative energy in and around you, there becomes a concentrated amount of only positive energy in order to heal your nervous system, decrease your heart rate, and increase your dopamine levels.

The way this works is by helping you to become one with the highest vibration of your energy, which balances your chakras and various centers, which puts your entire being into alignment. It does so by allowing your energy to flow freely without restrictions, being encumbered, or reroutes. It is like if you are driving down the street and there is a detour: you are going to have to use more fuel in order to follow the new path, rather than your original one. Blockages of your chakras make your life energy do the same thing.

While we may experience benefits from always being technologically connected, it also means we are being stimulated at all times, sometimes even while we sleep! This can, and often does--even without you knowing--lead to sensory overload, which is a completely exhausting experience. It triggers the most basic, animal survival instincts that you have, and it tells you that you are under attack. And if you think about it, you sort of are! Because you believe you are now in survival mode, it activates lots of responses in your body, brain, and energy that just are not necessary for your average day-to-day life.

When you are in fight, flight, or freeze mode, your body goes into autopilot. Your heart starts beating faster, breathing becomes more labored, restricted, and shallow, your muscles start to tense up, your body temperature rises, making you sweat, and your adrenaline starts pumping. While all of that turns on, many of your bodies' other functions actually shut down or slow to a crawl, because they are less crucial to your absolute survival in the moment. And all of this just because you got a notification on your phone! While these responses are necessary and important in the event of emergencies, to have extended periods of time living in this state is unhealthy and takes its toll.

Imagine all the energy your body expends reacting physiologically to that kind of stimuli, and then multiply it by the number of times you hear an alerting kind of sound--your phone notifications, breaking news, car horns, even your alarm clock. That is a lot of energy directed outside of your central flow of chakras, and away from a balanced self.

Using Reiki to alleviate stress is the lifeblood of the art of healing, putting the nervous system back into a state of normal functioning, allowing all the parts of your body and energy to reset to their original, unencumbered purpose. This slows your heart rate, slows your breathing, and allows your lungs to fill more expansively, providing more oxygen for your bloodstream, turning off your adrenaline, and releasing your clenched muscles.

Often times, stress will manifest itself in certain areas of the body, so some helpful areas of note include: the forehead where we furrow our brow, the stomach where we get knots, the neck and upper back where we scrunch our shoulders up, and the ribs where we hold our breath. Focusing our Reiki energy to these areas will not only help to alleviate the stress we are holding in our body, but it also helps to untangle the energy blockages that happen in these areas, as well as making a mind, body, energy connection with these areas, which help us to recognize these symptoms in the future, creating a level of consciousness that we will be able to more quickly address.

Reiki's success in assisting with relaxation and stress reduction is so pronounced that many hospitals even include it in their services. The art of healing by laying of hands is that special extra care that health professionals can use to increase recovery rates and maximize patient appreciation.

Anxiety and Depression

It is not just basic levels of general or acute stress that Reiki has been proven to assist with. It is also a complimentary service to treat more intense feelings of anxiety and depression. Of course, with more serious cases, Reiki should not be used as the only form of treatment, but many doctors suggest using Reiki in conjunction with their other forms of healing regimen.

While anxiety is a form of and a result of stress, it is different in quite a few ways. It often manifests itself in the form of sleeplessness, being irritable, irregular heartbeat, chest tightness, sudden feelings of fear, nausea, feeling out of control of their emotions, and headaches. The thing that classifies it as anxiety is its recurrence on a frequent basis that allows it to disrupt your regular life.

As we discussed in earlier chapters, Reiki is especially important in helping to eliminate worry. While worry and anxiety are different things, they are related, and therefore Reiki will be a logical solution to the more elevated, exaggerated, and overwhelming version of anxiety. Keep in mind the second rule of Reiki, "Today only, I will not worry." Worrying is a mindset that you can control, and although it may seem automatic, that is only because you have not yet mastered the ability to stop yourself short and redirect your thoughts. Much like worry, anxiety is your mind and body telling you that something is not right and that you want something to change. While you may not know exactly why or what it is that is causing your anxiety, you do not need the source in order to treat it with Reiki. In fact, the simple solution is to take action by using Reiki! Something needs to change, and it could be something as simple as focusing on your energy. That is a change! You do not need to try to push the anxiety out of your mind, as this will only make it stronger and more powerful because it gets to live in the shadows and mystery. Instead, you can simply redirect your thought from how overwhelmed you are feeling to allowing your own energy to wrap around, though, over, and under those anxieties and let them melt away. This may take some practice before it becomes an automatic trigger, but over time it will become easier and more automatic.

Depression is a deep feeling of sadness, loss of interest in your regular activities, and a general sense of hopelessness. It can be acute and brought on by a specific experience and last for a relatively short amount of time, or it could also be an ongoing chronic form that follows you through most of your life. This is not simply a bad attitude or wrong mindset. Depression is a very real, serious, common, and treatable condition that actually changes the way your brain actually works.

As discussed in chapter five, Reiki has many benefits to our mental health, which is why it is so successful in helping to relieve anxiety and depression. The flowing of energy does not just work on a superficial level, but rather on a deep level within your internal mood. By clearing your energy blockages throughout your body, it will help to release any stored up negative energy that could not escape before. It also brings positive energy in its place, helping you to heal yourself emotionally. This will bring yourself back to your Universal source center within your body, it aligns your chakras, which allows your heart and soul to flow freely to all parts of your body and mind. It lets your natural love seep into your whole self, as well as radiating outward to others and all the world's beings.

Giving yourself the love that has been restricted or lacking will help break the illusory patterns that have tricked you into thinking that you do not deserve the love or positive energy that you or the world has for you. When you are able to reignite that loving energy within yourself, it will also allow that same energy to come through you from the outside world.

Studies have shown that Reiki has offered benefits for many aspects of treating anxiety. It has been shown to lower people's stress levels, increase relaxation, improve mood, and assist with sleep quality. Research has determined that women especially found a decrease in anxiety in comparison to those who did not use Reiki. They also found that it works especially effectively for older adults for both anxiety and depression.

Physical Pain and Illness

Perhaps the most astounding effect Reiki can have is on physical pain and illness. Because this art is not fully understood scientifically at this point in time, many people are skeptical of its viability.

However, its results have been proven and speak for themselves. Beyond just clearing our soul and mental health, Reiki absolutely can help physical manifestations of our pain and illnesses. It is about reminding your body that it has the energy to heal itself, so when you follow that logic, it actually makes perfect sense that it assists in the physiological presentation of symptoms. The amazing thing about Reiki is that it does not require that you--or anyone else--understand or believe in it for it to work.

The list of ailments that Reiki has helped with is endless, but includes:

- Joint pain
- Muscle pain
- Chronic pain
- Migraines
- Nausea
- Fatigue

- Infertility
- Digestive issues
- Irritable bowel syndrome
- Crohn's Disease
- Heart disease
- Cancer

Of course, just like with anxiety and depression, Reiki should not be used alone as the sole source of treatment for any physical ailments, but it has been proven to help complement other medical treatments in all sorts of cases. That being said, the reason it is so successful in complementing Western medical practices is because it is a more well-rounded and holistic approach. Rather than just addressing the physical manifestation of the pain, Reiki focuses on the energy of and surrounding that issue. That pain you have been experiencing does not only live in that exact spot. Your entire body has been affected by it, and the energy in and around it has been blocked restricted, and changed because of it. In the same way that neurons transmit messages from your body to your brain, Reiki transmits that same information, but on a grander and more soulful level. So if you have not treated the energy around the pain, it is more likely to linger or return.

Many people arrive at Reiki to manage pain as a last-ditch effort after every medical and drug solution has failed. However, it has been shown to be most effective in conjunction with traditional treatments, including physical therapy, chiropractors, massage therapy, exercise, and acupuncture, among others. By allowing the energy in your body to flow unencumbered throughout all parts of you, this will help to heal all elements of your body that need it. Putting yourself in a healing mindset allows your muscles to relax and release the tension they are holding onto, allowing for free range of motion in joints, increased oxygen flow, and sending messages to your brain that the area is becoming free of impediments.

The best part of all of it is that there are no negative side effects attributed to the use of Reiki! Because the Universal life force is all-knowing, your body will only take in what it can accept, and therefore the Universe will never give more than you can handle. There will be no alternative pains or overdosing associated with Reiki as a pain management treatment. In order to do so, the practitioner will use a few different techniques in order to maximize the effectiveness of the session, such as clearing out negative energy, infusing the area with positive energy, centering you within the Universe, beaming healing to the areas in need, aligning your chakras, as well as smoothing out your aura. Not only does all of this encourages your own energy systems to heal themselves, but it also assists with more traditional medical treatments by preparing your body for their treatments, making those even more effective.

Because physical manifestation of pain, injury, disease, and illness is reflective of the energy happening in your body, it only makes sense that part of healing should include cleansing and aligning the energy throughout your centers. Part of the work of Reiki in relation to treating physical symptoms is focusing on the specific chakras associated with the area or source of malady. For instance, any pain or illnesses related to the lower body, addictions, and immunity issues are usually associated with the root chakra, so the Reiki practitioner will transfer a lot of cleansing energy through this location. The navel chakra is tied to hip, reproductive, and low back imbalances. Most issues surrounding digestion, the liver, diabetes, or fatigue are connected to our rib cage chakra. The chest chakra affects many huge areas of concern, such as lung and breathing problems, heart problems, and breast cancer. Unsurprisingly, the throat chakra is associated with issues around jaw and throat pain, glandular issues, thyroid problems, and even scoliosis. Concerns around brain and neurological issues are linked with our eye chakra. Finally, the chakra on the top of the head is associated with exhaustion and all physical disorders that manifest themselves without a clear source.

There are countless studies that show the results of Reiki are as effective as other forms of treatment. One study proved that Reiki is as effective at increasing range of motion as physical therapy, improving the muscles and joints of the affected areas. Patients reported that they required less pain medication than their untreated counterparts. It also assists women who have undergone C-sections during childbirth, women who have received hysterectomies, and patients who have underdone colonoscopies in managing their pain, anxiety, blood pressure, and breathing. Many hospitals across the United States have begun including Reiki as part of their treatment plans, especially for patients dealing with cancer. It is great at relieving the symptoms associated with it, especially fatigue, pain, depression, and quality of life. For this same reason, it has been shown to increase white blood cell production, improving the immune system. In fact, Reiki may be more effective at reducing fatigue than even meditation!

Chapter 14: Levels Of Reiki

Before getting started with Reiki, it is important to know that it comes in different levels or degrees. They can be seen as rankings, much like how an employee can go from a low-level position to a high-level one in their respective field. You can also see them as a way for an individual to upgrade their skills, going from beginner to intermediate until reaching the advanced level.

3 Levels or Degrees of Reiki

In the world of Reiki, there are three levels or degrees. When one is interested in practicing Reiki, you will need to climb these levels to master the healing methods. They will especially come in handy when you want to see what goes beyond the current level you are in. Such degrees also represent a person's ability to fully understand Reiki healing. This is a way for the student to become a master in the end.

First Degree

The first degree or Level 1 of Reiki is a practitioner's initiation. It is open to everyone and has the goal of helping individuals to be comfortable with the Reiki principles. This is where you will learn the ins and outs of the practice, as well as how it works right from the start.

The students who wish to become practitioners in the near future will have their attunement in Level 1. Done by the Reiki masters, the attunement will help them connect to the life energy that surrounds us. Previously, it would have been done in four separate sessions, but you only need one to complete it these days.

Also, it is known that students going through Level 1 will be given lessons about Reiki's history and methods along with group practice sessions.

In a way, the first degree encourages practitioners to take the first step towards mastery.

Second Degree

The second degree or Level 2 allows you to practice Reiki on others while making use of the symbols and slowly expanding or opening more energy channels. This is where the student will begin to apply what they have learned from Level 1 and share their energy to others. They can also understand what the symbols mean and how they can be utilized while practicing Reiki.

Level 2 helps practitioners learn new techniques of channeling energy, such as the method of being able to draw the symbols and send healing energy to others even when they are in the same room.

As for the Level 2 attunement, the intensity is quite high since this is where the student will begin to open the central channel. That's why Reiki masters have recommended to wait for at least 21 days up to three months before trying to jump from the first level to the second one. Once the waiting time is over, the students at Level 2 can undertake the attunement process.

Another thing to take note of the Level 2 attunement is that the Reiki symbols for power, harmony, and distance are given to a student by the Reiki master to indicate that they are finally being passed onto them.

It is not common, but it has been said that some Reiki masters even combine the lessons of Level 1 and 2 together.

Third Degree (Inner Master)

Finally, the third degree or Level 3 of Reiki represents a student's mastery. Known as the Inner Master, the student becomes the teacher at this point. Mostly referred as a Reiki master, this is when they can become the practitioner.

By reaching Level 3, the student will not only learn more methods but also gain the opportunity to attune others. In this way, the newly-appointed master can pass on what they have learned to help others achieve their goals as well.

The Level 3 attunement, commonly referred to as the Master Attunement, will have the practitioner open up energy channels on a much deeper level than what was achieved in Levels 1 and 2. To put it in a simpler way, it is where the session will get more intense than usual. Just like in Level 2, one must wait for a while before undertaking the Level 3 attunement.

With all this being said, it is important to remember that not all of the Reiki masters teach the same way. Even when they are practicing the Usui Reiki method, they may add some moves and guidelines that are not seen in the traditional way. So, make sure to do your research and pick the Reiki master whom you feel will bring you closer to your goals.

How to Ascend Through Reiki Levels

Unlike other alternative healing methods, ascending through the levels or degrees of Reiki healing has a process. First, when you have learned what you need to know from Level 1, you must go through an attunement process with a certified Reiki master who has already achieved the highest level. Second, you will take courses that will help you achieve the succeeding levels. This means you will study the lessons, practice methods, and understand other essential things that will assist you along the journey. You will also learn the distinctive points of the levels and how vital they are when mastering Reiki and integrating the symbols.

Once the time passes after your Level 1 attunement, you can undertake the Level 2 attunement. After that, you will become a Reiki master by the time you achieve Level 3. This is where you will tackle your master attunement task and become recognized as a real practitioner. From there, you can help others who would like to achieve the same thing and give them their attunement as well. You can even put up your own practice and become a practitioner like the other Reiki masters across the globe.

Keep in mind that when you are ascending through the Reiki levels, you need to be patient and observant. You cannot rush through all of them at once. Instead, take your sweet time and let yourself be one with the process. This will also give you a chance to apply what you have learned and practice everything. It will come in handy when you start learning the new healing techniques later.

Remember that your journey doesn't end even when you become a Reiki master. At Level 3, you will see that it has only begun. More opportunities, pathways, and experiences await you now.

Chapter 15: Reiki Stones

What are Reiki Stones?

Reiki, specifically, is the system of healing that believes, in using conduits, powerful, precise intra-universal life force energy may be utilized to create healing effects. This energy is commonly referred to as prana, mana, chi, source, and Holy Spirit.

This energy helps to promote healing effects in all types of living things on the material realm, as well as the mental, spiritual, and emotional levels. This energy may be utilized to heal nearly any type of ailment with nothing more than the sheer force of universal energy. In using this energy, all the true organic medicine may be better achieved without the use of even the most natural products.

More specifically, Reiki uses Ki, which is natural life force, to heal. This uses non-physical life force to alter the life force of an individual to create healing in some fashion. Using Reiki allows for the body, mind, and spirit to be healed simultaneously.

How does Reiki work?

Reiki may be used for everything that needs healing in some capacity. Some healers even are able to heal ailments that have not yet presented themselves yet, or emotion issues that lie in a person's past. It all depends on the ability of the healer and his or her understanding of the art of Reiki. It has been known to heal serious and life-threatening problems such as the flu, heart disease, sclerosis, and even cancer, but it also is able to heal minor problems such as colds, cuts, scrapes, broken bones, headaches, sunburns, insomnia, fatigue, sore throats, poor memory, impotence and even the lack of confidence.

The treatment basically fells like a warm light passing through your body, as it progresses, cold areas of the body are warmed. Those cold areas represent different ailments in the body that need healing. Thus, Reiki may be used to forgo negative side effects of western medicine, shorten healing time and eliminate pain.

Reiki utilizes Reiki healing stones that have individualized markings cut into them. These marking represent a specific type or style of healing for an individual healer. These stones act as a conduit from raw spiritual energy to the body. It cleanses the aura in the body by clearing out negative energy in the chakras. It also helps diminish doubtful or untrue thoughts about oneself to better achieve spiritual awareness. In clearing out the negativity, the body is able to better function and extract negative materials with the new energy granted by the healer.

Just by clearing out the chakras, the raw energy is able to heal even the most severe ailment. In this way, Reiki may be used on any person of any religion, or any plane of spiritual thought. All people have these chakras, thus, all people may be susceptible to the healing power of a Reiki stone and a Reiki healer. Reiki's healing power is more than just the reliving of symptoms, it is the actual, true healing of the potent negative energy that corrupts the body and effectively kills a certain part of the spirit by clogging the chakras. All that Reiki truly does is free the chakras so that the body is whole.

Reiki is an ancient art that has been used for several thousand years. With its healing power, most any ailment, large and small, may be fully healed to the core.

ABOUT CRYSTAL HEALING REIKI

Reiki treatment is considered a form of spiritual energy healing, which is believed to be guided by the vast intelligence of the universe, or Universal Life Force, that which we have come to know as the mind of God.

Crystal Healing Reiki is widely used by many Reiki healers. Their use aids in the balancing of energy within the body which in turn helps in the therapeutic process. Reiki practitioners use crystals because they can speed up the healing.

The purpose behind laying crystals or gemstones is basically to aid in the releasing of physical, emotional, spiritual or mental blocks. It is believed that negative experiences, both physical and emotional, can cause blocks in the energy paths which in turn bring about disease.

The gemstones are laid on specific points of the body where the chakras or energy centers are located. The practitioner's role is to be comforting, non-judgmental, and supportive making the patient feel "safe" in case he feels the need to release his emotions verbally. In many instances, the healing begins once the patient feels the freedom to express himself. This is an integral part of the healing process.

Reiki healers seem to have a preference for quartz, since it is a clear and harmonically shaped crystal, which properties apparently clear the blockages within the body. However, since chakras are associated with colors according to the energy fields they represent, many practitioners will take this into consideration when choosing the crystals to be used during treatment.

It is believed that these crystals have unique vibrational energies connected to their color and shape. This seems to help in the balancing, realigning and amplifying of energy fields within the body. It is important to always use a stone that feels good to the patient when placed on his body. If any discomfort is felt, the crystal should be removed at once. A variety of stones can be used and interchanged during treatment, and once the patient has 'absorbed' the energy from one stone, it should be removed. For this to be effective, the practitioner and the client must work closely together during this process.

The gemstones should be cleaned and kept in optimal conditions so they keep their energetic properties. Thus, after treatment the gems should be placed in salt water, and some Masters recharge them through specific techniques.

The following are some of the crystals used for Crystal Healing Reiki:

For the pelvic area, onyx, garnet and ruby can be used. The colors that represent these chakras are brown, black and red.

For the abdominal area, tiger's eye, quartz and amber are used. The color associated to this area is gold.

For the Third Eye or forehead, moss agate, amethyst and sodalite are indicated. The colors of this area are dark blue and purple.

For the throat area, turquoise, aquamarine and amazonite are indicated. The colors associated with this area are light blue or blue green.

For the crown or top of the head, quartz is used. The color of this stone is clear white.

For the heart area, pink tourmaline, rose quartz, rhodonite, aventurine, and green tourmaline can be used. And the colors associated are pink and green.

For the solar plexus, stones like malachite, peridot, rhodochrosite and moonstone can be used. The colors of this area are coral and chartreuse.

Chapter 16: Reiki Massage For Stress Reduction

Reiki has turned out to be an exceptionally powerful pain and stress management tool for me over the past three years. The real incident that Reiki assisted me with was because of an auto collision where I was back finished at a stop-sign, the other auto was traveling at around 30 mph and slammed my vehicle into the auto in front (also stationary). Luckily, there were no broken bones, just soft tissue harm. However, because of having von Will brand Disease, I (in the same way as other of you) couldn't take the calming prescriptions to help with recovery and because of my own sensitivity to pain solution, was relying on Tylenol versus more grounded analgesics.

The whiplash from the mishap required active recuperation. The scope of movement enhanced over two or three months of PT however the pain was still intense, so I looked for the assistance of Dana Young, an expert Reiki practitioner. The main session yielded recognizable pain help and strength relaxing, the following sessions continued to diminish the pain and increase the time between the fits. After two years, I have what the orthopedic specialists would call an interminable neck pain. Once in a while I'll take Tylenol to facilitate the pain if a fit goes ahead, however I realize that a Reiki session will dependably be more powerful long haul; helping my body to mend rather than cover manifestations.

The following is a depiction of Reiki from the Master Reiki Practitioner that I've seen for the past 3 years, Dana Young of Dragonfly Reiki:

Reiki is a relaxing light touch therapy that assists the mind and body in returning to its common condition of parity. Clinical perception and some preliminary confirmation from little studies show that Reiki treatment can be gainful for:

- stress alleviation
- Anxiety and sadness
- Pain, discomfort and other palliative consideration
- Insomnia
- Digestive issues
- improved heart rate variables in cardiovascular patients
- Side impacts from tumor treatment, including queasiness and exhaustion
- Recovery from surgery or games injury
- Overall well-being.

Definitive benefits connected with Reiki treatment are to feel healthier and more content and advance toward a condition of more prominent mindfulness. These ideas are like other types of Eastern-based medicine and mind/body works on, including meditation, Tai Chi, I Gong, yoga, acupuncture, Traditional Chinese Medicine and shiatsu.

Reiki is anything but difficult to learn as a practice for self-care and adjust. Self-treatment is particularly useful for people undergoing treatment for health issues, or who live with incessant health conditions.

Reiki treatment is a strong tool for use as a supplement to customary medicine, and is increasingly being offered in numerous hospitals, restorative consideration and therapeutic settings. Reiki treatment ought not to be a substitute for general therapeutic consideration from a qualified professional.

As a physically dynamic individual, my body is pushed really hard. With the riskier sports like snowboarding where a fall could prompt terrible bruising or broken bones, I take insurances by using Humane-P beforehand (and obviously wear a head protector!). However, if an injury is a sprain, muscle pull or other type of harm that may take more time to recuperate, I go to Reiki to facilitate the pain and energize healing. Reiki has been a protected, viable pain management tool that might be a possibility for others. While choosing a practitioner make certain to check qualifications, get referrals and so forth pretty much as you would a physical therapist.

Stress Relief

Stress has different causes and can be investigated from different points of view.

From a physical point of view, stress causes blood to hurry to the extremities, and empowers the apprehensive, endocrine, and resistant frameworks. While there is a possibility that the fleeting impacts of stress may be extremely valuable, on the off chance that we experience a tiger for instance, the short and long haul impacts of stress in present day life are to a great extent simply adverse. A straightforward Google hunt will give us a not insignificant list of the diseases and disorders brought on by respective stress.

From a passionate point of view, stress happens on the grounds that we feel that we are at some level, incapable of handling a situation. Nature implied for stress to help us in life-threatening situations in the wilderness. We don't live in the woods any longer, and it is just when we intentionally or intuitively see a situation as a risk, that we feel stressed.

An understanding of our vitality frameworks will show us that stress is just conceivable when our vitality bodies are feeble. A few parts of cutting edge life, for example, traveling, television, PCs and the internet, computer games, garbage sustenance, and so forth prompt in increase noticeable all around component in our bodies. This implies every situation influences us profoundly, leaving us powerless to stress, and dejection and an absence of association with our friends and family.

At the point when people come to us for a transient arrangement, we help our customers by working on these levels. Reiki is scientifically turned out to be compelling in stress diminishment and management, in reducing the circulatory strain and rate of heartbeats and boosting the safe framework. We utilize hypnotherapy or vitality work to offset the feelings and the vitality bodies, strengthening a man's resistance to stressful situations.

For a long haul answer for stress, it is best to learn and hone Reiki on oneself. Reiki enhances physical health and passionate and mental agility, which enhance your proficiency at work, as well as increase the level of quiet one experience in day by day life.

Chapter 17: Three Pillars Of Modern Reiki

The Three Pillars of Reiki are: Gassho (Gash-Show), Reiji-Ho (Ray-Gee-Hoe) and Chiryo (Chi-Rye-Oh).

Gassho

Gassho signifies "two hands meeting up". Gassho holds the aim of appreciation, regard, center, parity and association to collective awareness.

The Gassho hand position helps centering and calming the brain during contemplation. Place your hands in praying position with your eyes closed and carry attention to the tip of the middle fingers.

In a seated posture, place your hands in Gassho position.

Concentrate on where your two middle fingers meet.

Give your contemplations a chance to diminish.

Discuss the 5 Reiki principles out loud or in your brain

Once you're done, express the intention of appreciation.

If you consider this reflection useful, it is advised that you perform it in the first part of the day and night for 15-30 minutes, in a perfect ambience for one month. You may think that it's important to keep track of your encounters, in order to reflect just as how your life circumstances change with time.

Reiji-Ho

Reiji signifies "sign of the Reiki control". Ho signifies "techniques". Reiji-Ho consists of three short rituals that can be performed before each Reiki session.

Lift your hands in Gassho position, before your heart. With eyes shut, request the Reiki energy to course through you.

Request the mending and prosperity of the beneficiary. Lift your hands to your third eye and request to be guided to where the Reiki vitality is required.

Allow your hands to be guided. Disconnect from any doubs you may have regarding the result of the session and trust the Reiki vitality and your instinct.

Chiryo

Chiryo signifies "treatment". Chiryo is performed by the professional holding their predominant hand over the customer's crown chakra and holding up until there is a sign to move, which the hand pursues. The Reiki expert keeps on utilizing their instinct considering the hand position until they feel the calling, as part of the practice.

The body and cognizance are associated by breath. We take in oxygen for physical survival and universal life power to feed and purge our soul.

Two of the shorter reflection rehearses:

Joshin Kokyu-ho is a useful breathing strategy for diminishing your pressure and refining your brain and body. It is likewise an incredible contemplation for both purging and healing.

Start in a to standing or sitting situation with hands in Gassho position. Close the eyes and inhale gradually, through your nose. Relinquish any pressure.

Hold your hands up as high as you can and envision the light (Reiki) showering into your entire body.

As you exhale, imagine that the light rounding your body is spreading out in every way, present and past.

Playing out this contemplation normally will reinforce your connection with Reiki. Some individuals, additionally discover that it increments their intuitive capacities too.

Dan Tian

The Dan Tian is situated in the belly between the navel and pubic bone. The Dan Tian holds a supply of vitality. By setting aside some effort to interface with this vitality point, you can expand your imperativeness and guarantee you are a reasonable channel for Reiki vitality.

Carry your psyche to Dan Tian and tune in to your relaxing.

While you are breathing in, imagine that white light (Reiki) is filling your head and travels down the focal point of your body into the Dan Tian. Between each breathe in and breathe out, the light spreads to all pieces of your body. Feel that the healing procedure is continuing.

As you breathe out, picture that the light rounding your body is spreading out everywhere.

However, Reiki is an antiquated type of Japanese healing that is polished by numerous experts around the globe. There is a supreme energy that offers life to each living thing and the Japanese call this "Ki." It is otherwise called Chi by the Chinese, Prana by various Asian societies and most of the western countries refer to it as the Holy Spirit.

Chakras, a Sanskrit language word signifying "wheels of life," are vitality focal points found all through the body. The situation of every one of the major chakras relates with an endocrine gland or organ controlling hormonal balance. These Chakras are situated at the base of the spine (root chakra), between the pubic area and the navel (sacral chakra), two or three inches above the navel (sun based plexus chakra), the focal point of the chest (heart chakra), center of the neck (throat chakra), in between the eyebrows (third-eye chakra) and top of the head (crown chakra).

Chakras speak to explicit parts of the cognizant being and their primary capacities and attributes are the following:

Root chakra

Color: Red

Body Parts: Adrenal organs, kidneys, lower area of the spine, leg bones.

Capacity: Grounds you physically.

Awkwardness: Afraid of life, confused, narrow-mindedness, inclined to savagery; low back, feet and leg pain.

Sacral chakra

Color: Orange

Body parts: Gonads, prostate, reproductive system, spleen, bladder.

Capacity: Deals with imagination, sexuality and feelings.

Irregularity: Overuse of substances, sex or liquors; sexual or regenerative issues; perplexity, desire and confidence issues.

Sun based plexus chakra

Color: Yellow

Body parts: Pancreas, liver, intestines, stomach, spleen, autonomic sensory system.

Capacity: Intellect and it is known as the source of individual power.

Awkwardness: Insecurity about monetary issues; need to control others; stomach related issue.

Heart chakra

Color: Green

Body parts: Thymus, heart, lower lungs, circulatory system, skin, hands.

Capacity: Bridge between the physical and spiritual Universes; center of spirituality, prosperity and love.

Awkwardness: Sad sentiments, dread, outrage and possible coronary illnesses.

Throat chakra

Color: Blue

Body parts: Thyroid gland, throat and jaw areas, lungs, vocal strings.

Capacity: Communication and mental inventiveness.

Unevenness: Communication breakdowns, excessive eating and drinking to keep away from reality; respiratory ailments, dental issues and low confidence just as outrage, antagonistic vibes and hatred.

Third-eye chakra

Color: Indigo

Body parts: Pineal gland, lower brain, left eye, ears, nose, focal sensory system.

Capacity: Intuition and special insight;

Awkwardness: Fear of dreams, cerebral pains, sleeping disorders, tension and discouragement.

Crown chakra

Color: Violet

Body parts: Upper brain, right eye.

Capacity: Direct association with soul.

Awkwardness: Loneliness, need to compare ourselves with others, fear of death.

By putting the hands over the seven Chakra points that are encountering any of the lopsided characteristics reminded and performing Reiki, these Chakras can be rebalanced, prompting wellbeing.

REIKI AND CRISTALS

Accompanying Reiki vitality with Crystals makes them a powerhouse in mending your physical, spiritual and psychical body by accelerating the healing procedure.

Utilizing mending stones when performing Reiki makes an astounding joint of energy! They are incredibly compelling and, when put together, they work in concordance to enhance healing possibilities. It is accepted that the association between the stones and Chakras will restore the Chakra into a sound vibration, along these lines mending the part of the body more effectively.

Reiki

Reiki Therapy has been around for many years and is known as Universal Life Energy. It has been perceived as coursing through every living thing and it's accepted to adjust our vitality stream and healing from inside.

Created by Mikao Usui, Reiki is utilized for the adjusting and blending of energies. It is most usually utilized in a type of treatment, from one individual then to the next to reestablish spiritual, physical and profound prosperity. Reiki can likewise be utilized to adjust the energies of creatures, plants, items, water and sustenance and so forth.

Benefits deriving from Reiki

• Promotes Harmony and Balance;

• Accelerates the body's self-mending capacity;

- Dissolves vitality limits and advances characteristic harmony between psyche, body and soul;

- Assists the body in purifying itself from poisons and supports the safety system;

- Aids better rest;

- Helps to diminish stress and anxiety;

- Enhances positive energy;

- Lifts mind-set and clears the psyche.

Precious stones

Precious stones convey certain energies and when they connect with our individual vitality fields or chakras, they can have a positive effect to boosting our prosperity and fitting our energies. Certain crystals help interface the vitality to our Chakras, which are vortices of life vitality. They work to associate the physical and spiritual components of our body.

Advantages of Crystals

- Help in bringing abundance and clarity;

- Boosting vitality levels;
- Help us in not 'giving up';
- Promoting energy;
- Help to associate personality, body and soul;
- Help to counteract sickness.

Picking a precious stone that speaks to you...

Here are only some healing precious stones and their implications, find their properties and what they could help you with.

AMETHYST

Gives unwinding, quieting properties. Allow amethyst's vitality of satisfaction to sooth away any burden that keeps you up during night. This precious stone works with the third eye and crown chakras. Amethyst encourages your body to have sound rest and unwinding and works with your third eye to offset the brain with wise answers for issues.

AMAZONITE

Assuming your psyche is contaminated with dangerous cynicism, tidy it up with Amazonite. Severe mental distress we may have encountered in our past creates vitality obstructions in our present and this can translate in communication difficulties, problems when it comes to seeing someone or even in your work life. By filling your throat and heart chakras with cherishing vitality, this precious stone helps to open you up, to discharge what has harmed you so you can get rid of your issues.

PYRITE

Generally known as "Trick's Gold" for its likeness to genuine gold, Pyrite is a magical fortune. As it helps in drawing in wealth and abundance, it is additionally accepted to hold a solid defensive energy. The intelligent idea of pyrite is something other than physical with its capacity to demonstrate to you which practices might keep you down, which make you increasingly mindful of what you have to change so as to vibrate the aim of abundane on a similar recurrence as pyrite.

ROSE QUARTZ

Potentially one of the most prominent mending precious stones! 'See the world through rose tinted glasses' by taking advantage of the love of rose quartz. This stone opens your heart chakra to each sort of adoration that you need: love, fellowship love, familial love, love for humankind or sentimental love. As a flush of bliss, sympathy, pardoning, harmony and clearness beats through you, rose quartz will help you in discharging poisonous feelings so your soul can at long last be free of cynicism.

TIGER'S EYE

This crystal's capacity to initiate fierce concentration and basic power reflects its tiger-like appearance. Tiger's eye moves your standpoint so you can increase a more profound comprehension of yourself. Is there a piece of you that you need to analyse? Another leisure activity you might want to try? An answer for an issue you haven't considered? Something you need to do or see? Tiger's eye interfaces with the sun based plexus and sacral chakras to give you the power to seek these callings.

SUNSTONE

Similarly, as the sun carries life to all the living things on Earth, Sunstone will revive your innovative soul. It advances vitality, inventiveness and imperativeness. Its radiating vitality helps you to remember the delight in making and motivating. Sunstone supports the sacral and sun based plexus chakras to breed certainty, power and initiative. Free from underneath the cover of self-question, your innovativeness will at long last thrive with the intensity of the Sun.

SMOKY QUARTZ

This gem doesn't have the sort of vitality that is going to give you a chance to sit in a dim, dull room and sulk. Smoky quartz will assist you with getting up, attract the blind to positive light and open the windows to give the demeanor of antagonism a chance to get out. Working with this lovely gem helps you defeat negative feelings, for example stress, desire, dread, outrage and even sentiments of wretchedness. Elevating your mind-set with this stone encourages you to stay adjusted and positive in any circumstance.

RHODOCHROSITE

The self-esteem precious stone that will battle sentiments of deficiency, lifting your spirit and giving you a mindset of self-esteem. You deserve the adoration you get and Rhodochrosite energy causes you to acknowledge that by topping you off with affection and delight for yourself. This gem of strengthening works by injecting your heart chakra with the fortitude and inspiration to take on new challenges. Give unequivocal love a chance to overwhelm any sentiments of bitterness

Conclusion

The next step is to get out your calendar, schedule exactly what time you will have your daily Reiki practice, decide exactly where you will be having your daily Reiki practice, arranging that space in order for it to be most inviting and ready for your practice, and then simply doing it.

The only thing that is stopping you from harnessing all of the vital energy in the universe in order to heal yourself physically, mentally, emotionally is your own attitude and actions. You can start right this very second to change your life if you are willing to be open to the original life source that is flowing through and around you right this very moment.

Please feel free to highlight and bookmark specific pages in order for you to refer back to them easily, as it is perfectly fine to need to refer back to this book during your practice. As you become more comfortable and routine in your daily Reiki practice, most of these will become second nature to you. Until then, you can always come back to reread the different sections as you need them and as they become more applicable to your Reiki practice.

www.ingramcontent.com/pod-product-compliance
Lightning Source LLC
Chambersburg PA
CBHW072010070526
44583CB00015B/1411